Fazil Alyev

Markers and role of the vagoinsular and enteric systems

Fazil Alyev

Markers and role of the vagoinsular and enteric systems

ScienciaScripts

Imprint

Cover image: www.ingimage.com

This book is a translation from the original published under ISBN 978-3-659-88586-0.

Publisher:
Sciencia Scripts
is a trademark of
Dodo Books Indian Ocean Ltd. and OmniScriptum S.R.L publishing group

120 High Road, East Finchley, London, N2 9ED, United Kingdom
Str. Armeneasca 28/1, office 1, Chisinau MD-2012, Republic of Moldova, Europe
Managing Directors: Ieva Konstantinova, Victoria Ursu
info@omniscriptum.com

Printed at: see last page
ISBN: 978-620-6-76357-4

TABLE OF CONTENTS

1. Introduction

Combined severe craniocerebral injuries are the most urgent medical and social problems of our time. Intensive scientific and technological progress, high speed of means of transportation, annual growth of the rhythm and pace of life in developed countries has sharply contributed to the increase in the negative dynamics of the frequency and severity of combined injuries [1,4,6,10,24,25,29,33,41,45,53,61,73,96].

According to accurate statistics from the World Health Organization, 45% died of their injuries at the scene, 12% during transport, and 43% in hospitals [14,15,61,90,216,224,241,256].

Relative to individual traumatized participants (^1.5-2%) when receiving combined injuries, high mortality rate (≈28.6%), lack of activity of organs and systems, as well as complication of the condition of already seriously ill patients is the cause of a secondary serious complication, resulting in a high percentage of mortality rates clearly proves the relevance of this problem [37,38,46,78,79,79,92,95,109,113].

The presence of high mortality rates in combined injuries relative to conventional injuries has attracted even more attention in recent years from scientists working in this field as well as practicing physicians [5,45,48,72,93,117,124].

Usually combined traumas consist not only in the total volume of injuries of various organs. It is a complex of complex laws and characteristics of pathological processes belonging to particularly severe specific categories, resulting in disruption of the activity of organs and systems. In this connection, not only resuscitators, but also surgeons, traumatologists, anesthesiologists and other physicians specializing in different fields of medicine are involved in the treatment of such seriously ill patients [21,26,61,72,91,113,114,119].

In combined injuries, along with the failure of the complex treatment process, early prevention of complications occurring in organs and systems in such injuries and treatment also face a number of difficulties. Therefore, both of these unanswered questions facing clinicians are inherently evaluated as an urgent problem waiting to be solved [11,14,15].

One of the important problems waiting to be solved is to find out the causes of acute erosion and ulcers complicated by bleeding in the gastrointestinal system at different stages and periods of the treatment process at combined severe craniocerebral traumas [17,20,21,26,28,37].

In combined severe craniocerebral trauma, the occurrence of acute erosions and ulcers in the stomach and duodenum system, complicated by gastrointestinal bleeding, exacerbating the course of the disease, aggravates its prognosis, which is the cause of an increase in the mortality rate. It is impossible to design and prepare effective preventive and treatment measures without accurately studying the pathogenesis. One of the problems associated with gastrointestinal bleeding is the possibility of occurrence without any signs of a more important disease. Despite the statistical data that on the background of major diseases complication of bleeding with acute erosion and ulcers is" 1421%, in fact due to asymptomatic cases their rates are higher (25-30%). Usually in 80% of cases of acute erosion and ulcers are complicated by gastrointestinal bleeding. Only 20% of complications of acute erosion and ulcers are accounted for [76,82,83,100,110].

In spite of the modern level of complex therapeutic measures at complication of bleeding by acute erosion and ulcers, the rates of lethal outcome remain high (30-40%). From this point of view, the occurrence of acute erosions and ulcers in the stomach and duodenum, their prevention and treatment of bleeding complications are the problems facing clinicians, which have not lost their urgency and importance of their solution [46,59,65,78,122,265,286,297,298,309].

In combined severe brain injuries, as a result of the effect of sudden strong stressor factors on the body, depending on individual characteristics, violations of mutual communication and balance in the gastrointestinal tract, sympathoadrenal, adrenocortical, vagoinsular and enteric systems, becomes the cause of macro-microscopic and ultrastructural changes in the activity of the stomach and duodenum and mucous membranes. Despite certain improvements in the study of polyetiologic mechanisms of changes in the gastrointestinal system, the severity of the disease and in various combinations of vagoinsular, enteric systems, hemostasis indicators, the role of hypoxia usually going in the pathology are not fully studied [11,15,25,64,64,91,91,207,210,222,229].

Hormonal factors mainly specifically at the level of cell and tissue metabolism: and sympathoadrenal - adrenocortical hormones, cardiovascular, vagoinsular and enteric enzymes influence the digestive system. The sympathetic components of the vagoinsular system ensures the production of high acidity in the fundic gastric region, which in turn ensures a consistent entry of enteric regulatory peptides into the blood system[55,63]. It is highly probable that the course of dynamics of these mechanisms and the dependence on the periods of the disease are disturbed in combined severe brain injuries.

When bleeding complicates acute erosions and ulcers, the disease is aggravated for a long time, and against this background the chance of death is high. As noted by intensive care specialists, it is very difficult to predict the impact of the formation of acute erosions and ulcers in the gastrointestinal tract during treatment on the course of the underlying disease [17,20,27,98,98,106,232,241,253,293,315].

In combined severe craniocerebral traumas, as the main factors in the formation of acute erosion and ulcers in the stomach and duodenum and in their complication with bleeding there are dominant causes and in the dynamics of the complex of these causes are closely interrelated. But which of the above factors plays a more important role in the dynamics of ultrastructural, cytohistologic, enzymatic changes in the mucous membranes of the gastric and duodenal system has not been fully studied and there are no sufficiently specific data about it [27,37,46,63,71].

At the same time, the violation of the limit of equilibrium between the medium and defense functions of the gastric and duodenal mucosa during the formation of erosions and ulcers their relationship with the rheological features of the blood have not been fully elucidated [68,69,85,95,251,260].

Due to the fact that patients with combined injuries arrive at the clinic in a very serious condition, then from that moment clinicians direct their attention to the treatment of the main disease and early complications (shock, intoxication, infection, hemorrhage, restoration of the activity of organs and systems), acute erosion and ulcers and prevention of their complications are forgotten or simply relegated to the background. Only manifested at different stages of the disease factors of acute erosion and ulceration, or their complications with bleeding attract the attention of clinicians. Severe changes occurring in organs and systems are further aggravated by bleeding, deep deficit in the body of plastic and energetic materials provides acceleration of these changes [116,117,122,124]. It is for this reason that the conducted complex of treatment in the majority of patients is not effective. Continued bleeding of acute erosions and ulcers increases the chance of death of patients [109].

About the frequency of acute erosion and ulcer formation in combined severe trauma, literature sources are also contradictory [83,90,187,247].

The dynamics of the effects of vagoinsular and enteric systems on the gastric and duodenal mucosa and on enzyme synthesis, as well as the presence of passing without symptoms of erosion and ulcers due to the failure of endoscopic and pH-metric examinations, the lack of accurate statistical data on this shows that the issue is not fully studied [95,97,99,101,105,129].

Examination of erosions and ulcers in patients with combined severe craniocerebral traumas, or not conducting a series of endoscopic and histologic studies of mucous membranes after their detection or conducting them at certain stages is a clear confirmation of the lack of a comprehensive solution to the problem [40,104,109,171,191,236].

Most endoscopic and pH-metric studies applied up to that time were usually performed after erosion and ulcers were complicated by bleeding. Due to the lack of regular investigations during the course of gastric and duodenal mucosal disease, no detailed information is available on subsequent changes in gastric acidity [110,113,117,124,266,293,308,310].

Differentiation of acute erosions and ulcers in the stomach and duodenum, histologic examination, macroscopic appearance, in some cases (in bleeding) final endoscopic examination, but the assessment was mainly given by the results of pathological-anatomical autopsies [8,11,39,53,56,58,58,61,71,71,94,97,97,108,118,129,230].

Occurring stasis on the mucous membranes of the stomach and duodenum, disorders in capillaries, at different (catarrhal, phlegmonous, gangrenous-necrotic) stages of inflammation gastric acidity, rheologic features of blood, vagoinsular and enteric systems, degrees of intoxication and hypoxia, connection with periods and severity of combined trauma with hemodynamic parameters have not been fully studied and the problem remains relevant [100,110,122,224,228].

Although the literature we reviewed in recent years has provided various statistics on the incidence of acute erosions and ulcers, they do not fully encompass a common understanding of the entity [65,78,82,113,230,284,315].

In patients with combined severe trauma with resulting acute erosion and ulcer in the stomach and duodenum, a joint study of the role of a complex of polyethiopathogenetic factors, the development of a new modern complex of methods of prevention and treatment is extremely necessary.

2. Current characterization of combined injuries

Global scientific and technological progress in society (development of chemical industry, construction of skyscrapers, introduction of high-speed technology into production, natural disasters, etc.) poses important medical problems for people [68,72,79,91].

In addition to the positive aspects of development, catastrophic changes in the nature of accidents, negative factors such as polymorphism of injury severity and combinations have brought clinicians face to face with serious issues. One of the problems of the inevitable scourges of modern times is combined injuries [98,113,114,151].

During automobile accidents, the momentum of a car moving at a speed of 110-120 km per hour≈ 0 when hit by a person whose weight is ≈70 kcis changing its momentum, when pointing in the opposite direction from the previous direction:

$P_K - P_H = mV_K - mV_H = 0-70$ kg x (30 m/s increasing in the direction of the initial momentum) = 2100 N-second

This change in momentum creates a continuing force for≈ 2 seconds.

Thus, this force

$$F\Delta t = 2100 \text{ N·sek} \quad F = \frac{2100N \bullet san}{2san} = 1050 \text{ N}$$

becomes equal.

The subsequent impact of objects hitting a person, their stiffness and flexibility play an important role in the distribution of this force and the severity of injury. Using the brakes of the car to reduce speed ¼ of a second the impact force on a person weighing 70 kg at the moment of impact is

$$F = \frac{m\Delta \upsilon}{\Delta t} = 70 \text{ кг} \cdot 4 \text{ m/cек} \cdot \frac{1}{1/4san} = 1120 \text{ N} \quad [70].$$

The effects on the body of concussive factors and on the nature of injuries during a fall from height are correspondingly slightly different. When a person weighing 70 kg falls from a height≈ 30 m

$$P = m\sqrt{2qh} = 70 \cdot \sqrt{2 \cdot 10 \cdot 30} \approx 1750 \text{ N}$$

Contact with an object during a pulse≈ 0.28 sec.

Gets an impulse with a force $F = \frac{\Delta P}{t} = \frac{1750}{0,2} = 8750 \text{ N}$

In both cases, by presenting the pathologic changes created by such forces, within a short period of time on the systems of the whole body, we confirm our opinion that combined injuries consist of very severe pathologic combinations and that the problem is urgent.

Combined injuries do not simply consist of the sum of injuries to different organs. They are separate processes of specific categories having their own features and laws. Thus, the main factors of receiving combined injuries are modern high-speed automobile accidents, large-scale destruction, falls from heights, powerful explosions, etc. and there are no standardized templates in the tactics of treatment of such patients [98,109,114,117,119,151].

Combined craniocerebral injuries are the most common type of combined injuries in mechanical impacts along with craniocerebral injuries characterized by the involvement of other organs (without the skull) [73,81,99,103,107,113,157].

According to literature information among the combined injuries, combined craniocerebral injuries account for 89.4%. Thus, combined craniocerebral injuries in combination with limb injuries≈ 44.8%, with pelvic bones 12.7%, with vertebral column 7.8%, with abdominal cavity 11.4%, and other combined injuries account for 9.5% [78,79,95,113].

Intercombination relations in combined injuries dominated by craniocerebral injuries are observed in the range: between musculoskeletal and abdominal organs 7.8%, musculoskeletal and thoracic injuries 3%, and thoracic and abdominal injuries 0.5%.

Despite the diversity and polymorphism of combinations and degrees of severity of combined injuries, craniocerebral injuries predominate among deaths (32.7%,) [78,79].

It is known that in combined injuries, the percentage of mortality is≈ 17.6% with limb injuries, 16.9% with chest injuries, 14.1% with pelvic bone injuries, and 3.1% with spinal column injuries[48,78,79,113].

The seriousness of the position of combined injuries is that these injuries to the body and other organs (chest, abdomen, head, limbs, etc.) are not their components. From the point of view of pathophysiology, combined injuries are a pathological process of a completely different quality and the injury of any other vital organ separately is fundamentally different from them. And therefore, unlike light injuries of two or more organs on the course of pathological processes and because of the general reaction of the organism, combined injuries with their features create serious problems for clinicians [9,16,24,25,29,34,43].

Thus, in combined severe traumas, changes in respiration, general blood circulation, disturbances in the circulation of liquor and organic changes in the brain, are the cause of insufficiency of vital functions and blood circulation of the brain. At the same time, violations of the entire metabolic process, oxidation-reduction reactions cause serious damage to the activity and substances of the brain. As a result, the need for oxygen in the brain and other tissues increases. Hypoxia and metabolic disturbance, in turn being the cause of respiratory center disturbance and brain edema, increases brain edema and motor excitation. And the latter, being the cause of increased impulses in fractured bones and other foci of pain, causes secondary shock and fat emboli. By fractures and loss of blood there is a deficiency of cerebral circulation. Disruption of protein, alkaline balance, and water-salt balance can lead to renal failure [6,36,43,45,49,53,59,62,91].

Thus, there is a vicious circle: damage to the brain, causing deterioration of the nervous regulation of the metabolic process, becomes the cause of violation of the entire metabolism, damage in the chest and abdominal cavity organs more deepening this process, create additional conditions for the violation of the vital activity of the brain.

And although the brain has features of strong self-regulation, these possibilities are not unlimited. A drop in blood pressure by 70-60 mmHg, disrupting cerebral blood circulation, becomes the cause of first functional and then morphological changes [36,48,79,92,95,184].

In patients with severe combined craniocerebral injuries in 7595% of cases in some degree due to the center of origin of vomiting is aspiration, which eventually due to aspiration pneumonia leads to serious complications.

Aspiration pneumonias, forming edema-inflammatory changes in the bronchial-alveolar system and complicating gas exchange, lead to hypoxia. Eventually disruption of the general and cerebral circulation, cerebral edema, stasis occurs in the mucous membranes of the stomach. Within the brain, the increase in cerebral edema disrupts the dynamics of brain, liquor and blood balance [36,48,52].

Disruption of any link in the chain in the triad results in disruption of the vasomotor and respiratory center (Monroe-Kelly doctrine).

Both because of early and late complications, according to the nature, severity of injuries, and taking into account polymorphism and polyetiology of combinations of combined injuries, it would be reasonable to unite patients according to their features into the following groups:

1. Combined craniocerebral injuries with damage to the facial skeleton.
2. Combined craniocerebral injuries with limb and pelvic bone injuries.
3. Combined craniocerebral injuries with abdominal organ damage.
4. Combined craniocerebral injuries with organ and thoracic injuries.

There are many different combinations between relatively segregated groups and these are challenges that researchers and clinicians face all the time.

3- Neurophysiology of the digestive system

In the early period of trauma in injuries of central origin, as well as injuries to the skull base and pharynx, vomiting occurs as a result of exposure of the blood-filled stomach, which becomes the cause of adynamic and organic disturbances in the secretory and hormonal activity of the stomach and duodenum.

Vomiting - consists of the process of removing gastric secretions through the mouth and esophagus. The center of vomiting is located in the reticular information zone in the center of the medulla oblongata. And the main role is played by neurons of the dopaminergic reflex zone. At this time, duodenal secretions are bile mixture, and as a result of strong reflux back evacuation of gastric contents,changes occur in the environment and in the mucous membranes of the stomach and esophagus [34,110,113].

During combined severe craniocerebral traumas, along with damage to various brain areas, there is damage to hypothalamic-pituitary structures, and as a result of adrenocortical system activity, the development of processes of hypercatabolism and hypermetabolism occurs. Protein cleavage to meet the need for synthesis of biologically active substances important for reparative processes in the immediate posttraumatic period, hyperglycemia is registered mainly due to neoglucogenesis. Protein cleavage affects the reduction of albumin and globulin, ultimately to the formation of antibodies and impaired immunity. And hyperglycemia leads to an unpleasant neurologic prognosis. Under conditions of hypoxia, hyperglycemia causes the development of lactatacidosis, and also some of the glucosanine is converted into excitotoxic amino acids, leading to the development of cerebral edema. The central origin of gastric acid activity, vagoinsular and enteric systems, and forced nasogastric probing becomes the cause of gastric acid-alkaline balance disturbance, leads to atrophy of mucous membranes [110,116,119,124,130].

Central and intestinal failure, combined paresis become the cause of increased irreversible processes in the mucous membranes and smooth muscle fibers (on the gastrointestinal walls). Recent studies show that the use of H_2 blockers to protect the gastric and duodenal mucous membranes may lead to infectious complications in the lungs. Ultimately increased cerebral edema and hypothalamic-pituitary hypoxia, disrupts reticular formation regulation and vagus nerve innervation [36,87,111,116,126,140,169,207].

Regulation of the occurring disorders in combined severe trauma in the digestive tract, which has complex neurophysiologic regulatory mechanisms, is a very important and significant issue.

4. The role of hormonal factors in the pathogenesis of changes in the stomach and duodenum in combined severe craniocerebral traumas

The influence of stress factors on the human body in severe combined traumas, in this or that organ or system in the formation of any disease is undeniable role of various types of compensatory reactions, i.e. adaptation syndrome. The adaptation syndrome itself is not a pathological reaction; on the contrary, it is an important physiological defense reaction that is protective against damage [92,95,102,104,107,113,130].

Sometimes this syndrome, like all biological reactions always has an effective optimal effect. Whether the syndrome hormones are fully or relatively increased, or insufficiently and incompletely increased, it plays a major role in diseases of the stomach and duodenum.

Sometimes the lack of adaptation syndrome, plays a greater role in the formation of pathological processes than in the specific effect of the pathogenic agent, and gives the predominance of adaptation to disease [92].

The continuation of a state of short-term or long-term maladaptation leads to the onset and development of disease in the stomach and duodenum [91,92].

The negative nature of maladaptation plays a larger role than the subject's response to exposure to trauma.

It should be emphasized that in combined traumas in the first minutes and hours, the sympathoadrenal phase of reactions to stress naturally during a certain period of time being replaced by vagoinsular (hypoglycemic, hypotonic, anabolic) phases includes a complex of reparative processes. Reaction to stress, the predominance of this or another phase depends on the nature of the trauma and severity. Responses of the neurohumoral system can also vary depending on the individual characteristics of the organism, immune system, age and sex [92,107].

By examining urine throughout the day, studying the dynamics of excretion of catecholamines, corticosteroids and their metabolites, and their real assessment, it becomes possible to clarify the compatibility of the sympathoadrenal system with the nature of the injury [82,110,113,119,151].

In the initial moments of injury, increased adrenaline (relative to noradrenaline) secretion by the adrenocortical system (gluco- and meneralocorticoids), an unstable equilibrium plays a special role in altering the degree of tissue sensitivity to catecholamines [82,92,110,275].

Duration and increase of adrenaline secretion, reducing tissue sensitivity to insulin, has a serious effect on carbohydrate metabolism. Creating a "centralization" effect not only in the cardiovascular system, but also in the whole body, at the same time has an effect at the level of cellular metabolism.

By reducing peripheral glucose utilization by≈ 20%, it creates a hyperglycemic adrenal stressor (relative to noradrenaline) [83,110,113].

In appearance, patients have pallor, cold sweat, dry mucous membranes, etc.

This is followed by the onset of hypoglycemia of the vagoinsular phase of the stress response.

Exposure of the organism to the duration of stressor factors (several hours, days and more) causes depletion of catecholamines reserve and, being a compensator, activation of adrenocortical system - increase of cortisol level. And this, increasing sensitivity to catecholamines, in all metabolic processes causes a relatively stable deep rejection. Not only functional, but also structural changes occur in the transportation of glucose into cells [110].

Slowdown of hydrocortisone utilization of glucose at the level of the Krebs cycle, glucose-dependently stimulates gluconeogenesis, reduces RNA synthesis and ATP formation. As a result, protein-free atrophy, immunosuppression gradually develop [116].

Glucocorticoids in high concentration show a mineralocorticoid effect, which results in decreased demand [81,107].

So, the total effect of hydrocortisone is the slowing down of specific tissue functions, which is characterized by the tendency of metabolism in the direction of depletion of the stock of functions towards catabolism [36].

Disruption of the long-term and sustained utilization of glucose in the tissue is perceived by a marked response from the insular apparatus of the pancreas. An increase in blood glucose increases insulin secretion. However, the resistance to insulin created by hydrocartisone places a high demand on the insular apparatus. In a state of slowed protein synthesis, this demand is particularly strong. As a result, by increasing pancreatic insulin secretion, cell hypertrophy and hyperplasia are increased.

Unfortunately, outside the portal system insulin levels do not really reflect synthesized, because 50-90% of synthesized insulin is "washed out" in the liver. And this circumstance creates difficulties in determining the real secretion of this hormone. During the transformation of inactive proinsulin into insulin, C-peptide is released, which is a residue of 23 amino acids. This peptide does not carry a hormonal function and like insulin does not have high specific receptors (p). And therefore, in comparison with the dynamics of the relative increase in C-peptide concentration, the increase in glucose concentration in circulation outside the liver, shows itself as a response to the increase in hydrocortisone concentration and is an indirect indicator of increased insulin secretion [31,40,45,60,73].

Thus, the increase of C-peptide in blood outside the liver plays the role of a more accurate marker relative to weighted insulin and glucose levels: first in hyperinsulinemia, second in insulin resistance.

There is a close relationship between the functions of the insular apparatus and the parasympathetic part of the autonomic nervous system. Stimulation of the vagus from the pancreas increases insulin secretion, and insulin, stimulating the transmission of cholinergic impulses, shows the advantage of parasympathetic influence [81,82,92,119].

There are other peptides of the enterin system that have similar insulin activity to varying degrees. Performing several functions to varying degrees in the enteric compartment on insulin forms, which can be considered as a number of peripheral regulators (APUD- sistem - AmineprecursorUptakeandDecarbaxylation) [110].

One of these functions is glycemic level-dependent regulation of glucose utilization, and the other is together with other enteric system peptides (gastrin, gastrointestinal polypeptide ^^,cholecystokinin, vasointerstitial polypeptide (VIP), etc.), and consists of Vagus-independent regulation of gastric secretion [110,163,165,179].

The co-existence in the vagoinsular system of the effect of vagus nerve irritation and the effect of insulin on the digestive system in a regulation-regulation mechanism is important.

The latter effect in the vagoinsular vagal impulse system is determined by the degree of insulinization, and the effect of catecholamines is determined by glucocorticoid levels.

Naturally, only between nerves (sympathetic and parasympathetic) and hormonal components - with autonomic function - on the one hand adrenaline, glucocorticoids and on the other hand insulin act on the basis of the existing mechanism of antagonism. The hormonal components compete mainly at the level of cell and muscle metabolism.

Sympathoadrenal effectors affect the cardiovascular system, vagoinsular and digestive systems [92,110,313,314,315].

Thus, in the organism the main digestive reactions in the norm is the activation of the vagus reflex, i.e. sympathetic components of the vagoinsular system in the fundal part of the stomach become the cause of gastric secretion with high acidity. The acidic environment of chyme, affecting the mucous membranes of the upper part of the stomach, gradually provides the order of successive transfer of enteric regulatory system peptides into the blood.

And in combined severe traumas these successive links, due to strengthening, weakening and imbalance of this or that link, fall into an unfavorable environment. As a result, there is aggression in both metabolism and acid-base balance. Disorders of central origin, hypoxia, changes occurring in the hemostasis system, depressions in the immune system, exposure to products of hypoxic metabolism and catabolism and for other reasons, the creation of the ground for imbalance in the activity of the vagoinsular and enteric systems lays the foundation for future pathology and complications [6,17,18,22,25,26,33,34,34,37,42,43,62].

On the background of combined heavy traumas instantly due to the contusion of the whole organism as if there is a "total earthquake". As a result of chaos in the ordered rows of the defense system, the occurring discrepancies both in the acid-alkaline balance of gastric secretions and in the system of hemostasis, being the cause of stasis "stasis" in the mucous membranes, leads to the formation of primary edema - liquid tumor [92,110].

From the effect of acidic environment, regulatory peptides (antigens) entering the blood circulation in interaction with receptors causes free histamine in the submucosal layer (fixing on the membrane of fat cells, antibodies). Massive long-term exposure to acid (on mucous membranes) causing an increase in enteric peptides, an increase in sensitization activity leads to "total tolerance". Thus, autoimmune reactions against their enterins and primarily to gastrin lead to the formation of erosions and ulcers in the mucous membranes of the stomach and duodenum [16,22,31,53].

As a result of depletion of specific immune reactions, no less specific immunity, with a small specificity of movements towards humoral immunity leads, to an increase in the number of B-lymphocytes and circulating antibodies.

Circulating in the circulation serum antibodies and immune complexes consisting of regulatory peptides, losing specific immunity, provide antibody preparation against these complexes. In a subsequent step, circulating antibodies interact with antigens and enterin peptidamines of the gastric wall (mucosal and submucosal layers). The process, according to the size of the loss first of all in the corresponding enterin zone (gastrin zone), and then with the loss of specificity of antibodies, occurring directly in the cell membranes, in the mucosal and submucosal layers leads to inflammatory reactions - local lesions. That is, lesions occur even earlier in areas in contact with gastrin zones, which pass acids into the gastric cavity [110].

In the presence of high digestive - peri-digestive function in gastric secretions, the presence of a source of local necrosis leads to the formation of typical peptic ulcers (erosions and ulcers). The localization of erosions and ulcers respectively depends on the autoimmune response of the mucosa in different regions of the enteric system (gastrin system). Naturally, anatomical localization on the gastric wall in the gastrin region plays an important role [110].

Refluxes, vomiting of central origin, prolonged spasms disturb the trophicity of smooth muscles and mucous membranes. The release of duodenal secretions into the gastric cavity only due to the neutralization of hydrochloric acid in the gastric cavity gives the effect of a certain compensator. The entry of bile acids into the stomach, because of the increase in the conductivity of the gastric wall tissues, ensures the transfer of enteric peptides into the blood [104,108,110,116,140,175,181].

In combined injuries and their various complications, the diverse effects of the above factors in the formation of acute erosion and ulcers in the stomach and duodenum and their complications, manifest themselves depending on the period and degrees of severity of the disease.

5. On the principles of equilibrium of interaction and feedback of vagoinsular and enteric systems

In normal physiology, during and after a meal, the amount of gastric secretion increases under the influence of regulatory factors and this mechanism carries out additional three phases - cephalic, gastric and intestinal. The centers of secretory reflexes are in the intermediate brain, in the limbic cortex and in the hypothalamus. Excitation from here is transmitted to the stomach by vagus nerve fibers [98,110,138].

Excitation of the vagus nerve, which is located in the stomach, results in the secretion of acetylcholine. And acetylcholine

directly awakens the principal and enveloping cells and stimulates gastrin secretion from G-cells located in the antral region. Gastrin causing the strongest secretion of HCL is directed by blood flow to the enveloping cells. There are light gastrins having a heavy and short period with a long period of cleavage due to a period of semi cleavage. Excitation of the vagus nerve, also increasing the activity of histidine decarboxylase, increases the amount of histamines in the gastric mucous membranes. Here histamine, collecting in fat cells and in histaminocytes located in the projection of envelope cells, dramatically increases the secretion of HCL acid. There are stages in the intestinal phase of gastric secretion, first increasing due to the ingestion of new portions of product into the as yet unacidified environment of the duodenum, and then decreasing due to the acidic environment. The increase at first is due to the secretion of gastrin from the G-cells of the duodenum. And the penetration of chymic acid into the duodenal environment is associated with secretion of secretin, which decreases gastric secretion in its mucosa [116,179,187].

Referred to figuratively as the "abdominal salivary gland", the pancreas and its enzymes play a distinctive and indispensable role in regulating gastric secretion and the digestive process [110].

All these enzymes, being at first in an inactive form, only after entering the intestinal cavity, begin to revitalize. Synthesized in the ribosomes of acinus cells, they are stored in the form of zymogen granules. Their release is the main factor of cholecystokinin (pancreozymin) secretion, and a sharp increase occurs under the influence of secretin [110].

The secretion of enzyme-rich pancreatic juice occurs as a result of the joint activity of secretin, cholecystokinin and the vagus nerve. Full realization of cholecystokinin effect is possible only in cases of secretin presence and vagus nerve intactness. The sympathetic nervous system affects only the delivery of blood to the pancreas.

After exposure to severe trauma - severe stress, there is a serious imbalance in the current chain reaction mechanism in the digestive system, regulated by very complex principles of interaction and feedback. Normally, the stepwise regulated secretion of digestive juice for food intake is regulated by vagal nerve branches - vagoinsular (primary) mechanisms and enteric (downstream) mechanisms. Entering the gastric cavity food mass contributes to the growth of gastric secretion, and the increase in acidity of mucus, which performs the protective function of the mucous membranes -mucins. The entry of chymous acid with a portion of food into the duodenal environment regulates the decrease in gastric secretion and acidity until the neutralization process is complete. The increase in acidity in the gastric environment regulates mucosal secretion and plays a very important role in equilibrating the acid-gastric balance in the stomach [65,79,92,283,303].

The stress-response of the sympathoadrenal system over a period of time in severe trauma - contusions naturally progresses to the vagoinsular phase - stage [110,310,314].

The increase in the amount of adrenaline as an early defense response, and in the next stage the increase in adrenocortical system activity along with the determination of the degree of sensitivity to catecholamines draws attention to the lack of agreement and equilibrium between them. Adrenaline, by creating an effect and centralizing blood throughout the body, decreases peripheral glucose utilization and creates stressor hyperglycemia. In response, pancreatic insulin secretion increases and the vagoinsular - hypoglycemic stage begins [110].

The state of prolonged stress - shock leads to depletion of catecholamines and, as a result, being a compensator, leads to activation of the adrenocortical system - increase in the amount of cortisol. That, increasing sensitivity to catecholamines, creates discomfort for patients. The whole exchange of deep and relatively stable abnormalities marks the presence of structural changes in the transportation of glucose into the cells,

As a result of the cumulative effects of hydrocortisone, with increased catabolism and depletion of specific function stores, abnormalities are observed.

Prolonged and sustained impairment in glucose utilization leads to increased levels of insulin secretion to an abrupt insular response.

Activation of synaptic components of the vagus (vagoinsular system) leads to high acid secretion in the stomach, and acid chyme to gradual and consistent transfer of enteric system peptides into the blood. From the above, we conclude that two systems play an important role in regulating the activity of the stomach and duodenum: vagoinsular and enteric systems, which interact and complement each other.

The role and responsibilities of nervous and humoral mechanisms in the digestive system have been confirmed at the level of modern science. The activity of nerve regulation is realized by sympathetic and parasympathetic influences. There is certainly a gradient of distribution (nervous, humoral, local) among the regulatory factors [109,275,282].

The role of gastrointestinal hormones in the activity and humoral regulation of the food system is particularly large (Table 1).

Table 1

Hormones involved in regulating the digestive system

Hormones	Effects
Gastrin	Increased gastric and pancreatic secretion, hypertrophy of gastric mucous membranes, increased motility
Secretin	Increased pancreatic bicarbonate secretion, delayed acid secretion in the stomach
Cholecystokinin (pancreosimine).	Gallbladder contraction, increased bile secretion, increased pancreatic secretion, decreased gastric acidity, increased pepsins in the stomach, increased peristalsis of the small intestine
U1P (vasoactive intestinal peptide)	Relaxation of smooth muscles of blood vessels (decrease in A/D), delayed gastric secretion
Motilin	Increased gastrointestinal motility, increased pepsin secretion, protein synthesis
Gip (gastrointestinal peptide).	Reduces gastric acidity, decreases motility
Somatostatin	Inhibits the secretion of gastrointestinal glands and hormones.
PP (pancreatic polypeptide)	Cholecystokinin - pancreosimine, being antagonists, increase mucosal proliferation, is involved in carbs and protein metabolism
Bombesin	By releasing gastrin it stimulates gastric secretion, by releasing pancreatic enzymes: cholecystokinin - pancreosimin - neurotensin - pancreatic peptides.
Regeneracin	Improves the processes of regeneration - repair of mucous membranes. Reduces gastric acidity

In case of combined severe traumas on pathology in the central nervous system (the main dominant trauma), in accordance with periods and degrees of severity of traumas of nervous regulation, in accordance with the changes created in the digestive system, the dynamics of humoral factors changes. According to the degrees of compensation for these changes, the basis for pathologic changes in the stomach and duodenum is laid [104,183,204,210,234,256].

6. etiology of disorders occurring in the vagoinsular and enteric systems in combined craniocerebral injuries

In severe combined injuries, the resulting trauma to both the central nervous system (brain and spinal cord) and other organs and systems (musculoskeletal, thorax, abdomen, and their various combinations) results in prolonged shock and coma.

Prolonged hypotension (A/d below 60-70 mmHg), hypoxia and hypovolemia, high processes of catabolism and metabolism, pathological abnormalities of the immune system do not pass without affecting both the central nervous system and the nervous and humoral mechanism of regulation of the digestive tract[36,79,92].

The impact of the above complex factors, as well as formed on their background pathological signs (vomiting, duodenogastric reflux, filling the abdominal cavity with blood), as a result of operations in the chest and abdominal cavity, in the neurohumoral, adrenocortical, vagoinsular and enteric systems, on the background of combined traumas, in regulating and complementary hormonal systems creates a serious imbalance - chaos.

In the organism at the initial stage and at the last stages of combined traumas along with early pathogenetic factors (proponents of combined) at the level of local, organs and systems secondary (sanogenetic) reactions occur at the level of local, organs and systems in response to the first ones.

As a result of disruption of neurodynamic processes of regulatory functions in the central nervous system, in vital organs there are disorders of the immune system and physiological activity. Depletion of adrenal gland reserves, an indicator of antigen loading of immunocomponent cells, which provides the advantage of T-lymphocyte - suppressors in the peripheral circulation.

The occurred centralization of the general circulation (protection against shock hypotension) leads to the occurrence of "protective" reactions (spasm, stasis, sludge phenomenon) and local edema in the local-regional cycle [79,92].

Progressive cerebral edema, impaired general and regional cerebral circulation creates an imbalance in the neuroendocrine system.

Inadequate responses of the neuroendocrine system to injury, neurovegetative corticosteroid blockade can cause irreversible damage to adaptive processes and metabolic cycle.

Due to profound hypoxia, disturbance in glucose utilization, hyperglycemia, glucose cleavage by Krebs cycle, disturbance of hemostasis system, disturbance of acid-base balance of gastric secretion, as a result of reflux of bile ejection into the gastric cavity, serious imbalance in hormones of vagoinsular and enteric systems and motility of stomach and duodenum is created.

In soft tissue injuries of the neck and extensive hematomas due to contusions of the vagus nerve, disturbances in the vagoinsular innervation of the stomach are formed. When the stomach is damaged due to surgical interventions, as well as gastric hematomas as if a complete or partial vagotomy of the vagus nerve is carried out, eventually there is a decrease in the vagoinsular effect. In gastric mucosal injuries, the effect on secretory activity is not without influence [6,24,31,41,53,62,90,95,100].

Hematomas and contusions of the pancreas and so must respond to central combined hyperglycemia, secondary to being subjected to secretory and vector load, transforming for etiologic reasons, laying the foundation for the development of severe pancreatitis (reactive).

The abnormalities occurring in the hemostasis system, temporary hypotony lead to: in the mucous membranes and in the submucosal layer stasis - sludge phenomenon, forming edema, imbalance of vagoinsular and enteric hormones, and acid-base balance [81,82,103,104,107].

For the purpose of forced evacuation, gastric probing, leading to loss of gastric secretion, to reflux of duodenal bile secretions into the stomach, lays the foundation for negative abnormalities in the balance of the vagoinsular and enteric systems and in the effects of hormones.

A fall in blood O_2 enrichment (saturation) leads to a fall in cerebral oxygenation, ultimately an increase in cerebral edema, a disturbance in adrenocorticotropic hormone preparation and mineralocorticoid deficiency. The effects of this deficiency on metabolism and the vagoinsular and enteric systems play a pathogenetic role in the pathologic changes.

From the effects of prolonged shock, microcirculatory and hemocirculatory disorders along with accession to local edema, sludge phenomenon, complications in the form of stasis and thrombosis, together with coma, create disorders in higher nervous activity, deep abnormalities in the activity of internal organs appear. Otherwise, vital organs as kidneys, pancreas, adrenal glands etc. are the first to be damaged.

Hypo - hyperglycemic, states, along with the effects on metabolism, becomes the etiologic impetus for abnormalities - disturbances in the vagoinsular and enteric systems.

The formation of favorable conditions for the development of infections in the oral cavity, in the upper respiratory tract can lead to the penetration of infections in the stomach.

Optimal conditions for the development of Helicobacter pylori are formed (decline of barrier and immune abilities of mucous membranes). As a result, there are violations in the secretory functions of the stomach. With the detection of barrier functions in the mucous membranes, bile acids in the gastric mucosa, as a result of the reconstruction of mucin in the gastric mucous membranes and an increase in breakdown products (sialic acids), the balance of the processes of anabolism and catabolism of the mucous membranes is disturbed. As a result, the acidity of the environment in the stomach and duodenum increases and the amount of insulin, cortisol and gastrin gradually changes, the amount of gastrin increases. All factors noted at the end, creating an imbalance in the vagoinsular and enteric systems, lay the foundation for future pathology in the stomach and duodenum [125,172,204,237,252,272,292,308].

7. Results of endoscopic (FEGDS) examinations of patients from the main group with severe combined craniocerebral injuries

In patients from the main group the dynamics of endoscopic parameters differs from the observed group, 10 people from each group, the studies were carried out on the 1 -5-7 days.

Beginning in the early stages of trauma, bile refluxes into the stomach as a result of filling of the stomach with blood from the upper respiratory tract, combined with central vomiting. As a result of the cleavage of blood from the effects of the acids of the gastric contents, and from the effects of the vagoinsular and enteric systems, the excitation of the gastric mucous membranes results in the secretion of gastric juice of high acidity. As a result of the cleavage of microproteins within the mucosal gels of bile acids, the barrier function of the mucosa is destroyed. As a result, with the appearance of abnormalities in the acid-base balance, increases the strength of the aggressive effect. As a result of deep hypoxia and shock, as a result of microcirculatory disorders occurring in the mucous membranes with trophic, destructive changes in the course of the disease, along with polyetiologic pathogenetic mechanisms becomes the cause of the formation of acute erosions and ulcers. Hypertrophy of secretory glands, hyperplasia of barrier epithelium and course changes towards destructive, necrotic changes, local disturbance of blood delivery (microcirculatory disorders), as a result of increased aggressive effects of bile acids and gastric acid, forms acute erosion and ulcers.

At the early stages of endoscopic examinations due to the severe degree of shock and coma, microcirculatory disorders in the mucous membranes of the stomach and duodenum, edema and congestion were detected. In cases of combined combinations of abdominal cavity organ injuries, such disorders were dominant. The results of endoscopic examinations on the 1st day are shown in the photos below (1,2 and 3)

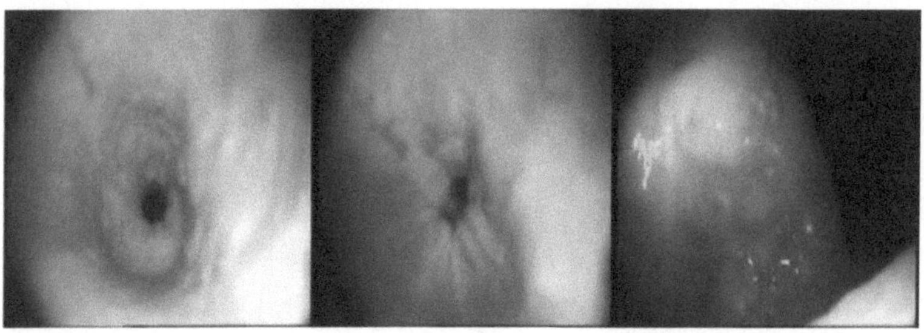

Figures 1,2,3. According to the combined combinations of acute erosions and ulcers detected on the 1st day.

In examinations on the 5th day of deepening inflammatory-destructive changes in mucous membranes, the presence of acute erosions is determined. The surface is covered with purulent plaque, which explains the transition of leukocytic infiltrative erosions in many areas into acute ulcers (Fig. 4,5,6)

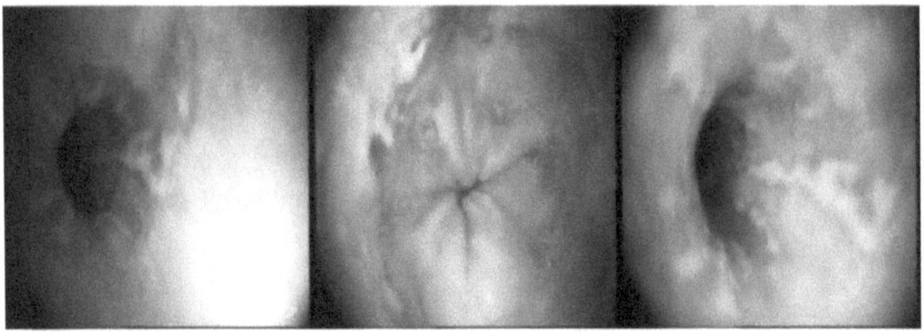

Figures 4,5,6. According to the combined combinations, acute erosions and ulcers detected on the 5th day of examination.

On the 10th day of examinations clear manifestations of already formed acute erosions and ulcers were determined by the presence of acid-hemotypic plaque on them (Fig.7,8,9)

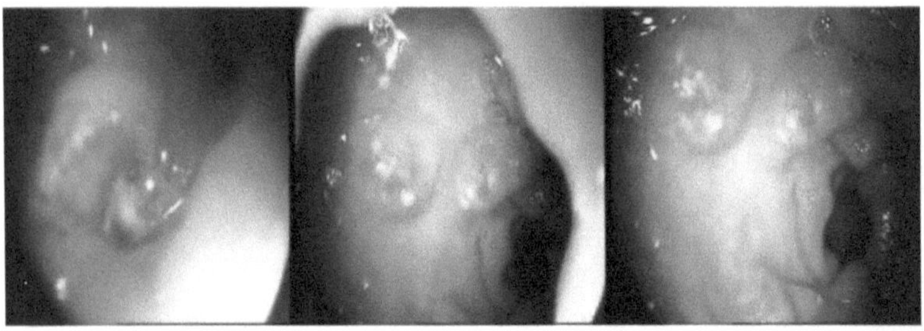

Figures 7,8,9. Corresponding to the combined combinations, acute erosion and ulcers detected on the 7th day.

Bleeding complications of acute erosions and ulcers were confirmed on the basis of gastric tube by the presence of precipitation of brown discharge or the presence of melena, and on the basis of blood examination.

8. Results of vagoinsular and enteric system examination parameters in patients with bleeding complications detected

In accordance with the goals and responsibilities of the examination of general patients from the main group, the dynamics of certain indicators of vagoinsular and enteric systems were investigated in patients with identified bleeding complications.

The results of the established indicators are given in the table below (Table 3.21).

In the 1-3rd day studies, the amount of insulin in the blood, being closer to the upper level of normal, including was close to the results of the general patients on the 5th day.

Table 3.21

Results of vagoinsular and enteric peptide indices in patients from the main group, with identified bleeding complications

(21 patients)

Resul-ts of research indicators	Days of surveys							
	1	3	5	7	9	12	15	18
Insulin µmv/mL	20,19±0, 93	20,11±0, 62	13,13±0,96***	11,11±0,57***	9,17±0,41***	8,23±0,37***	7,18±0,27**	6,91±0,2***6
C-peptide ng/mL	4,17±0,19	4,09±0,16	3,71±0,23	3,01±0,09	2,23±0,21	2,16±0,17***	4,91±0,11**	4,41±0,19
Glycosylated hemoglobin %	5,61±0,23	5,17±0,19	5,13±0,21	5,41±0,23***	5,66±0,23***	7,67±0,37***	6,71±0,31**	6,21±0,21
Gastrin pg/mL	121,33±4,51	121,17±4,19	111,13±4,12	91,17±3,11***	79,61±3,17***	76,43±3,51***	73,25±3,19***	70,53±2,13***
Histamine µg %	12,9±0,5	12,7±0,5	12,9±0,7	12,9±0,9	11,9±0,7	11,7±0,6	11,3±0,7	11,1±0,7*
Somatostatine ng/mg	K.5,7±0, 3 Q. 5,3±0,3	5,1±0,5** 4,9±0,1	4,5±0,3*** 4,2±0,2**	4,4±0,3*** 4,2±0,3*	4,3±0,3*** 4,3±0,2**	4,1±0,4*** 4,1±0,2**	3,9±0,3*** 3,3±0,2***	3,7±0,2*** 3,1±0,3***

Note: Staggered exact difference statistics with performance: Accurate difference statistics and 1st day performance:

* -p<0.05; ** - p<0.01; *** - p<0.001

C-peptide values are 10.4% higher than the upper limits of the norm. Being 13.5% lower than the upper limit of the norm glycolyzed hemoglobin began to correspond to the indicators of general patients on the 5-7th day.

The results of gastrin on this day, being 12.1% more from the upper limits of the norm, began to correspond to the general indicators of the main patients on the 3-5th day.

The histamine values, being 12.9% higher than the upper level of the normal limits, became consistent with the results of the general patients on days 3-5.

Somatostatin values, being 11.4% above the upper limits of normal, became consistent with the results of the general patients at day 15.

The amount of insulin in the examinations on the 5th-7th day, corresponding to the average values in the norm, being 15.4% lower relative to the early values, began to correspond to the values of the general patients on the 7th-9th day.

C-peptide values, being 13.3% below normal and 13.8% below normal on the first day, attracted attention. The glycolyzed hemoglobin survey values were below normal by 13.6% and early values by 10.9% .

In the studies of gastrin indicators, corresponding to the upper level of the norm, in comparison with the early indicators decreased by 13.3%. Histamine indices, being higher than the upper limits of the norm by 12.9%, were at the level of early indicators.

Somatostatin values were 11.4% of the upper normal range and 12.9% lower from early values.

In studies on days 9-12, insulin amounts, approaching the lower level of normal, were 24.5% lower than early values.

C-peptide values, while corresponding to the average level of normal, were 19.3% lower than early values.

Glycolyzed hemoglobin values, corresponding to the upper limit of normal, increased by 10.9% relative to early values.

Gastrin values were 12.6% lower from the upper limit of normal and 15.9% lower from early values.

Histamine values were 1.2% higher than normal and 10.8% lower than early values.

Somatostatin values were 11.6% of the upper limits of normal, and 13.3% lower than early values.

In examinations on days 15-18, insulin values, corresponding to the lower limit of normal, were 29.1% lower than early values.

C-peptide counts were 12.3% above the upper limits of normal and 11.8% above the early values.

Glycolyzed hemoglobin values, corresponding to the upper level of normal, were 11.9% higher than early values.

In histamine studies, it was found to be lower from the upper limit of normal by 13.7% and 16.6% lower from early values

Histamine values were found to be 1.13% higher from the upper limit of normal and 11.4% lower than early values.

9. Results of immune lysis and precipitation reactions in patients from the main group complicated by bleeding

In accordance with the purpose of the research work, the dynamics of observation of the studied indicators of immune lysis and precipitation reactions in patients complicated by bleeding was carried out in general patients from the main group. The obtained results are given in the table below (Figure 3.22)

In the studies conducted on the 1-3rd day, sialic acid values, being above the upper limit of the norm by 22.2%, remain high, as in the main group.

Protein C-reactive protein values, increased 2-fold from the upper limit of normal, were higher by 22.6% .

Table 3.22

Indicators of immune lysis and precipitation reactions in patients from the main group complicated by bleeding (21 patients)

research indicators	**Days of research**							
	1	**3**	**5**	**7**	**9**	**12**	**15**	**18**
Sialic acid in plasma mmol/L	5,17±0,2 1	5,33±0,5 1	5,13±0,4 1	4,17±0,3 1*	3,11±0,1 3***	3,27±0,1 9***	3,51±0,3 1***	4,17±0, 27**
C-reactive	13,3±1,1	12,7±1,1	12,9±1,3	13,1±1,1	13,3±1,3	13,5±1,2	13,7±1,0	13,7±1, 0
protein mg/l								
Antistreptolysin-0 (AEST) mv/mL	421,1±22 ,1	423,4±21 ,7	417,3±21 ,3	347,1±21 ,9*	331,3±21 ,3**	317,1±21 ,1**	297,3±21 *** ,3	261,1±2 ⅛⅛⅛ 3,3
Antihyaluronidase (AEyS) mv/mL	321,7±21 ,9	321,9±22 ,7	317,6±21 ,9	311,5±21 ,3	303,3±21 ,1	297,1±21 ,3	251,1±21 ,7*	247,3±2 2,7

Note: Accurate stepwise statistics of variance and performance:

Accurate statistics of the difference and performance of the 1st day:

* -p<0.05; ** - p<0.01; *** - p<0.001

Antistreptolysis-0 was 21.1% above the upper limit of the norm. Antihyaluronidase values were found to be 10.7% higher than normal.

The amount of sialic acid at examination on the 5th-7th days, remaining as high as on the first day, was 16.5% higher. In the same order, the C-reactive protein indices, being at the level of the first day, were 21.8% higher.

Despite a 12.1% decrease in 0-antistreplolysis relative to the first values, there was a 17.3% increase above normal.

Although a decrease of 10.3% was recorded in antihyaluronidase examination values relative to the primary day, there was an above normal 10.4% decrease.

In the study of 9-12 days, in the indices of sialic acid relative to the first day decrease of 15.8% , there is an increase of 12.9% of the norm.

Protein C-reactive protein indices, remaining at the level of the first day, were recorded above the upper limit of the norm by 22.5%.

As a result of the examinations, despite a 13.3% decrease relative to the primary indicators of antistreptolysis-0, it was found to be 15.6% higher than normal.

Antihyaluronidase values are 10.1% below the upper limit of normal, and a decrease of 10.8% is observed compared to the primary values.

In the study of indicators of 15-18th day was found sialic acid 12.4% below the primary indicators, but above 8.1% of the upper limit of normal; C-reactive protein, remaining at the level of the primary indicators above the norm by 22.8%.

10. Results of gastric contents examination of patients with bleeding complications

All patients from the main group underwent gastric content examination, the focus was on patients from this group with bleeding complication.

The results of the study are presented in the table (Table 3.24)

Table 3.24.

Results of gastric contents of patients from the main group with bleeding complication (21 patients)

Indicators under study	Days of research							
	1	**3**	**5**	**7**	**9**	**12**	**15**	**18**
gastric pH-ι	4,07±0,17	4,03±0,11	3,71±0,15	3,63±0,13*	3,57±0,13*	3,31±0,15"	3,67±0,15	3,73±0,11
Bile acid в stomach mq/l	0,52±0,03	O,51±0,01	0,48±0,02	0,51±0,02	0,52±0,03	0,52±0,01	0,51±0,01	0,47±0,02
Sialic acid в stomach mq/l	0,61±0,04	0,61±0,03	0,57±0,03	0,54±0,03	0,51±0,03	0,48±0,02"	0,42±0,03"'	0,41±0,03"'

Note: Exact stepwise difference and performance statistics: Exact difference and performance statistics of day 1:

* -p<0.05; ** - p<0.01; *** - p<0.001

Indicators on the 1-3rd day: relatively alkaline pH of the stomach, which is lower by 11.6% of the upper limit of normal. The amount of free sialic acid in the stomach is 20.3% higher from the upper limit of normal, and the amount of bile acids is 46.9% higher than normal.

Indicators on the 5-7th day: pH-1 of the stomach approached the upper limit of the norm; the amount of free sialic acid in the stomach in contrast to the first day decreased by 10.9%. Indicators of bile acids in the stomach in spite of insignificant decrease on the first day were 41.5% higher than the upper limit of the norm.

Indices on the 9th-12th day: gastric pH-1 at the upper limit of normal; free sialic acid in the stomach above normal by 17.4%, 11.6% lower from the primary results; bile acids in the stomach above normal by 36.9%, lower by 12.7% from the primary results.

Indicators on the 15th-18th day: pH continued to remain at the upper limit of the norm, however, relative to the primary result changed by 11.1%. Free sialic acids in the stomach were 14.5% higher than normal, 13.9% lower than the primary result; bile acids in the stomach were 31.5% higher than normal, 14.8% lower than the primary result.

11. Results of endoscopic examination (FEGDS) of patients from the main group who had bleeding complication.

In patients with bleeding, a nasogastric tube was inserted, gastric contents were aspirated and endoscopic examination was performed. During the study as a source of bleeding , acute erosions and ulcers were identified on the mucosa of the stomach and duodenum. A photograph of the detected acute erosions is presented below (Fig.10).

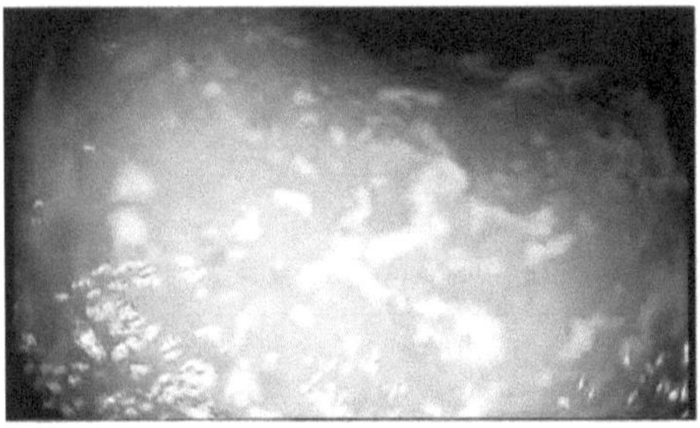

Fig.10 Magerramov R.A. VII

Gastrointestinal bleeding on day 14 of neuroresuscitation.

The bleeding due to acute erosions and ulcers and their localization, according to the results of endoscopic examination, were distributed among the combinations of severe traumas indicated in the table below.

Tab. 3.26

Dependence on combinations of combination , localization and cause of bleeding in patients from the main group (21 patients).

Causes and sources of bleeding	Patients with severe combined craniocerebral trauma and fractures of limbs and pelvic bones (3 patients)	Patients with severe combined craniocerebral trauma and abdominal organ injury (11 patients)	Patients with severe combined craniocerebral trauma and chest and lung injury (7 patients)
Multiple erosions in the stomach.		1(4,7%)	
Acute gastric ulcers		1(4,7%)	
A complication of chronic peptic ulcer.	1(4,7%)		2(9,5%)
Acute erosion duodenum	1(4,7%)	2(9,5%)	1(4,7%)
Acute erosions of the stomach and duodenum		1(4,7%)	1(4,7%)
Acute ulcer duodenum		2(9,5%)	1(4,7%)
Exacerbation of chronic ulcer duodenal ulcer	1(4,7%)	2(9,5%)	2(9,5%)

Note: Accurate stepwise statistics of variance and performance:

Accurate statistics of the difference and performance of the 1st day:

* -$p<0.05$; ** - $p<0.01$; *** - $p<0.001$

Status of vagoinsular and enteric systems in patients with gastroduodenal bleeding

For complex polyetiologic reasons, in patients with severe combined craniocerebral traumas, the formation of acute erosions and ulcers, complicated by bleeding, is observed on the 7-15th day.

Bleeding is usually accompanied by melena, or vomiting in the form of coffee grounds. In patients with a nasogastric tube, it manifests as bloody contents with coffee grounds. In blood tests, there are serious abnormalities in the hemostasis system, in the coagulation and anti-coagulation systems.

As a result of imbalance and barrier functions of the gastro-duodenal system, formed acute erosions and ulcers complicated by bleeding, blood pouring out of the stomach - duodenum cavity reacting with hydrochloric acid, forms a compound hydrochloric acid - hematine, which in turn irritates the mucous membranes, which contributes to increased secretion.

In contrary cases, when bleeding is accompanied by vomiting, there is abundant reflux of bile acids into the gastric cavity.

Being already in poor condition protective system of the gastro-duodenal system, as a result of imbalance between the factors of defense and aggression is subjected to even greater changes. Accelerates the process of cleavage of mucoproteins of the mucosal barrier by bile acids. High acidity of gastric juice increases the production of gastrin. At the same time, depending on the degree and intensity of bleeding, the reserves of adrenocortical, vagoinsular and enteric systems are used, which are aimed at stabilizing hemodynamics.

Against the background of blood loss, protein deficiency is formed and to maintain the balance, against the background of high catabolism, protein breakdown in muscles and gluconeogenesis increases. Due to relative protein deficiency, serious systemic abnormalities.

As a result of irritation of the mucous membranes (chyme with high acidity, bile acids, blood cleavage products), the activity of the vagoinsular system increases. Ultimately, the rate of transfer of enteric peptides into the blood increases (Fig. 4.4).

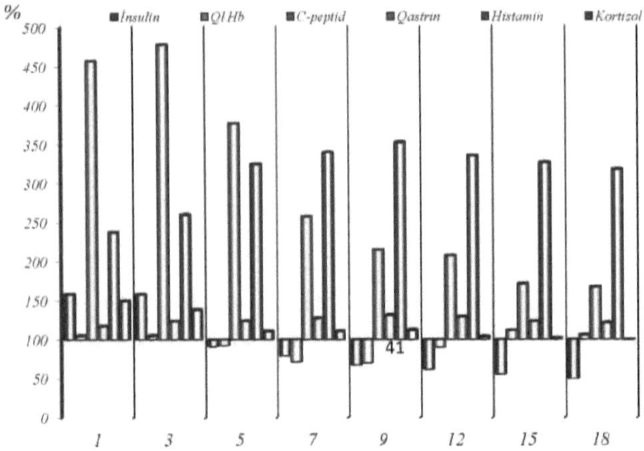

Fig.4.4 Activity of vagoinsular and enteric systems in patients of the main group (norm - 100%).

Bleeding against the background of acute erosions and ulcers, further exacerbate changes in the hemostasis system. In ulcer bleeding indicators of the antiplatelet system in the blood sharply increase, and this system together with the vascular - platelet reaction of the coagulation system, forms a vicious circle. In bleeding, the simultaneous increase in plasma and plasminogen activity, and the detection of FDM in the blood leads to even greater disturbances in the hemostasis system.

In the early days in the presence of bleeding, relatively unstable high indices of vagoinsular and enteric systems are noted. Starting from 3 - x days there is a dynamic decrease in these indicators. In the stomach, the indicators of bile acids and sialic acid increase. Simultaneously with the dynamic increase in gastrin, there is an increase in the concentration of histamine in the blood.

Indices of vagoinsular and enteric systems in hemorrhage, are summarized in the table below (Table 4.5)

Table 4.5.

The state of vagoinsular and enteric system parameters in gastroduodenal bleeding in patients from the main group (21 patients)

Indicators under study	Days of research							
	1	3	5	7	9	12	15	18
Cortisol mmol/L	384,17±13,13	381,13±12,17	367,19±11,11	358,17±11,21	351,19±11,09'	347,09±11,01'	341,14±11,03'	341,09±11,01'
Insulin µmv/mL	20,19±0,93	20,11±0,62	13,13±0,96'''	11,11±0,57'''	9,17±0,41'''	8,23±0,37'''	7,18±0,27'''	6,91±0,26'''
C-peptidng/mL	4,17±0,19	4,09±0,16	3,71±0,23	3,01±0,09'''	2,23±0,21'''	2,16±0,17'''	4,91±0,11''	4,41±0,19
Gastrinpg/mL	121,33±4,51	121,17±4,19	111,13±4,12	91,17±3,11'''	79,61±3,17'''	76,43±3,51'''	73,25±3,19'''	70,53±2,13'''
Histaminemcg %	12,9±0,5	12,7±0,5	12,9±0,7	12,9±0,9	11,9±0,7	11,7±0,63	11,3±0,1	11,1±0,3
Sialic acid in plasma kmol/L	5,17±0,21	5,33±0,51	5,13±0,41	4,17±0,31'	3,11±0,13'''	3,27±0,19'''	3,51±0,31'''	4,17±0,27''
Bile acids in stomach mg/L	0,61±0,04	0,61±0,03	0,57±0,03	0,54±0,03	0,51±0,03	0,48±0,02''	0,42±0,03'''	0,41±0,03'''
Somatostatin ng/mL	K.5,7±0,3 Q.5,3±0,3	5,1±0,5'' 4,9±0,2	4,5±0,3''' 4,2±0,2''	4,4±0,3''' 4,2±0,3'	4,3±0,3''' 4,3±0,2''	4,1±0,4''' 4,1±0,2''	3,9±0,3''' 3,3±0,2'''	3,7±0,2''' 3,1±0,3'''
stomach pH	4,07±0,17	4,093±0,11	3,71±0,15	3,63±0,13'	3,57±0,13'	3,31±0,15''	3,67±0,15	3,73±0,11

As shown in the table, on the 1 - 3 - e day during bleeding there is an increase in the level of cortisol in the blood. Increase in cortisol level, as a result of catabolism acceleration due to activation of vagoinsular and enteric systems increases the level of insulin and G - peptide in the blood.

By irritating the gastric and duodenal mucosa with highly acidic chyme and bile acids, leads to an increase in gastrin.

In the first 1-3 days gastric pH values are high, in the following days there is a dynamic decrease.

On the 1st-7th day due to the increase in the amount of circulating antibodies and gastrin, there is a high level of histamine in the blood. Due to the reflux of bile into the stomach, the breakdown of mucoproteins, which have a barrier function, is accelerated. As a result, the amount of sialic acid is high in gastric contents and plasma on the 1st-5th.

In the first 1-3 days, the concentration of somatostatin in the blood is high, but decreases in the following days.

Despite the compensatory "secondary" increase of vagoinsular system and enteric peptides on the 1-3rd day during bleeding, their amount decreases in the following days.

12. general principles of resuscitation and intensive care of patients with combined severe craniocerebral trauma

The modern concept of intensive care at the early acute neuroresuscitation stages of patients with severe combined craniocerebral trauma provides for the prevention of intracranial and external complications and stable control of the total intracranial volume, as well as the regulation of reperative and sanogenic processes of the central nervous system against the background of treatment measures. Adequate assessment of the condition of the injured at the first stages of trauma (1-3 - and day) plays an important role in characterizing the development of the acute period and preventing the probability of critical increase in intracranial pressure and secondary ischemic changes in the systems.

Functional monitoring with recording of early indicators plays an important role in assessing the effectiveness of treatment. The implementation of timely measures is a significant means of preventing the development of clinical signs observed in the sub- or decompensation phases. Functional monitoring provides an opportunity to determine the effectiveness and rationality of treatment.

Attention is drawn to the fact that the fatality rates for cases of severe general craniocerebral trauma are still too high. Attention is drawn to the severity of craniocerebral injuries, the degree of multisegmental damage, the exposure of the whole organism to shock and the existence of a direct correlation in the age of the patients. In questions of disease topogenesis, decisive role is played by decompensation of injuries, as a result of which immediate brain death becomes the cause of subsequent unmanageability.

The formation of the mutual complication syndrome plays a decisive role in the formation of the subsequent vicious circle for the organism. In such cases, there is always room for multiple opinions about unfavorable outcomes and disease progression.

It can be noted that some of them play a major role in limiting compensatory reactions during the response of the central nervous system and the organism as a whole.

Favorable conditions are created for the occurrence of secondary extracranial damage, and sometimes the cause of this is unreliable intensive complex treatment of organ and system injuries at the neuroresuscitation stage.

The direct connection of common brain injuries to other organs and systems further deepens the severity of brain injuries.

Depending on the localization of extracranial injuries, certain pathological syndromes may occur and develop. As a result of multifactorial analyses it became clear that for the confluence of complications with the main pathology at the primary stages of traumatic disease, in addition to the period of shock duration, the degree of shock, the volume of bleeding and blood loss, aspiration of food mass and blood into the lungs, massive chest injuries hypokinetic type circulatory disorders and hypertensive dislocation syndrome, the fundamental role is played by the implementation of additional infusion-transfusion measures. Failure to implement adequate anesthetic measures and sedation, repeated surgical interventions, retroperitoneal hematomas, traumatic pancreatitis, damage to parenchymatous organs, the development of purulent-inflammatory processes, fat emboli, failure to implement therapeutic and prophylactic measures to prevent the development of acute erosions and ulcers of the gastro-duodenal intestinal system.

In this regard, the main ways of optimal intensive care should be: ensuring the earliest possible regional and systemic perfusion, prevention of additional formation of intracranial damage, prevention of systemic disorders (systemic hypoxemia, hypercapnia and hypodynamia), early enteral hydration and nutritive nutrition, respiratory treatment, implementation of rational antibacterial therapy.

During the resuscitation period, treatment should be based on the following principles:

1. Ensuring adequate central perfusion pressure (CPP) by correcting hemodynamics. The main goal is to provide oxygenated blood to the brain. To enrich the blood with oxygen, the most effective means is STA. For adequate transportation of oxygen to the brain by blood, Hb should be maintained at least 100 g/L and Ht at least 31 -33%. At the same time, it is necessary to prevent thromboembolism. For this purpose, O_2T and O_2T enrichment in STA patients are carried out. In cases where blood pressure is low, adrenomimetics are used according to compatibility combinations. Noradrenaline (epinephrine) 1-2 ml with 0.9% Sodium Chloride solution 100 - 200 ml intravenously, or Dopamine 5 - 10 ml in solution in the specified volume, 60 drops intravenously are administered. Taking into account the specified critical limit of hypovolemia, erythrocyte mass or native plasma is transfused from of the same group. Taking into account hypercoagulability, as well as in order to prevent thromboembolism and fat embolism, Fraxiparin 0.3-0.6 units 1 ml is administered every 8 - 12 hours subcutaneously, as well as Lipostabil 10 - 15 ml with own blood intravenously.

2. In order to ensure the qualitative composition of infusion therapy and correction of electrolyte disorders, the increase in blood osmolarity should be carried out with the use of sodiumemia, glycemia and potassiumemia.

During infusion therapy, isoosmolar and slightly hyperosmolar crystalloids should be given preference. The volume of transfused fluid should be calculated in the amount of 50-60 ml / kg of weight. The exact volume of transfused fluid, and electrolyte equilibrium is prescribed according to the water-electrolyte balance disorders.

In critical situations, "capillary leakage" (loss) occurs due to impaired patency of microcirculatory veins. Administration of hypoosmolar solutions in the neuroresuscitation period is not recommended.

In infusion treatment, the basis of isoosmolar and slightly hyperosmolar crystalloids are solutions of Sodium Chloride; of balanced saline solutions - "Trisol" 50 - 60 ml / kg - g, in the volume of 500 - 600 ml / hour, as well as Ringer's solution in the same volume. In order to prevent "capillary leakage" as blood substitutes use a day of 50 ml / kg hydroxystarch preparations, resulting in improvement of the rheological environment and blood coagulation system (can be increased to 800 ml / day).

3. The goal of transfusion treatment is to restore the oxygen transport function of the blood and to correct disorders of the clotting and anti-clotting systems of the blood.

In order to restore the loss of hemostasis system it is recommended to use fresh frozen plasma in the volume of 200-250 ml. It is best to resort to this in cases when the prothrombin index drops below 70%.

In order to treat thromboembolism and DIC syndrome it is necessary to carry out heparin therapy from 4 - 5 days of the disease.

During the decrease of hemoglobin below 70 g/l in complications due to gastrointestinal bleeding in order to improve the supply of oxygen to the brain it is advisable to administer 750 ml of red blood cell mass daily or once a day.

In such cases, it must be remembered that there is a risk of acute lung damage after transfusion. If the results were relatively below the critical limits, fresh erythrocyte mass and native plasma were administered intermittently, respectively, based on the necessary instructions. The day after the blood transfusion, urine tests were obligatory.

4. Prevention and treatment of DIC. Fresh frozen plasma or cryoprecipitate are used to replenish losses of the blood coagulation system.

In addition to organ dysfunction, coagulopathic disorders can lead to other thromboses and embolisms. Low molecular weight heparin is used to prevent such events. A prophylactic dose according to the disease combinations is indicated from the first day of injury. Fraxiparin, reopolyglucin, lipostabil, trental are used as indicated. Daily hydrobalance: it is possible to control up to 50 ml.

5. Diuretics should be used with great caution by prescribing K^+ 2 times a day. Mannitol, Lasix, Spironolactone are prescribed for this purpose.

6. Sympathomimetics should be administered after or together with infusion drugs by means of

an automatic dosing device (perfuser or infusion machine). It should be used until the appropriate hypertensive effect of controlled blood pressure is achieved.

Each patient is treated individually and after elimination of internal bleeding, Noradrenaline and Dopamine are administered in necessary doses according to the age and weight of the patient.

7. Hypotensive agents. When brain injury predominates in joint craniocerebral injuries, there is a predominance of hypertension.

Increased blood pressure plays an important role in supplying blood to the brain. The use of hypotensive drugs lowers BP but has no effect on lowering intracranial pressure. In such cases, brain edema is not reduced and the risk of ischemia increases. Except for severe cardiac pathologies, the use of hypotensive drugs is not appropriate. Since the leading component of compatibility is brain injury, hypotensive drugs should be used with great caution.

8. Antiarrhythmic and coronarolytic drugs. The sources of the changes occurring in cardiac functions are mainly hypokalemia, hypomagnesemia and central nervous system disorders. If, due to the disturbances, cardiac arrhythmias dramatically lower blood pressure and heart rate, cordarone (amiodarone) may be used by infusion. In ventricular tachycardia, magnesium sulfate in the amount of 30 - 35 / mg / kg weight can be applied intravenously. In convulsive arrhythmias, a mixture of glucose+ calcium+ insulin is effective in 50% of cases.

Atropine (5 - 10 mcg/kg) or adrenaline (3 - 5 mcg/kg) may be administered during acute sinus bradycardia, sinoatrial blocks

In arrhythmias accompanied by hemodynamic disturbances, at the initial stage at intervals every 5 minutes administered cordarone 150 mg, at the subsequent stage at intervals of 2 - 3 hours - 300 mg.

Administration of cordarone 150 mg 2 times intravenously is called the "gold standard" of cardiopulmonary resuscitation for ventricular tachycardia. Of the coronarolytics, nitroglycerin and cardicert are used intravenously.

9. Ensuring the patency of the respiratory system. To ensure the function of the external airway, it is necessary to ensure patency of the nasal and oral cavities. These processes are carried out directly during tracheal intubation. The insertion of an intubation tube prevents the development of secondary inflammation of the brain by the unimpeded delivery of a mixture of oxygen+ air to the lungs. On the other hand, in this way we prevent microorganism-rich mucus from entering the trachea through the mouth and larynx. The indication for tracheal intubation is not only respiratory insufficiency, but also the brain. Therefore, intubation is recommended in cases with supportive breathing in order to prevent cerebral hypoxia. If necessary, intubation by tracheostomy surgery should be performed when indicated. Confidence in ensuring the patency of the respiratory tract was achieved by periodic

bronchoscopy.

10. Provision of external respiratory functions. In the neuroresuscitation approach, artificial ventilation (AV) is used for respiratory failure and brain failure. The mode of artificial ventilation should be carried out in accordance with the severity of pathology, modes should be selected accordingly. Periodically it is necessary to perform bronchoscopic sanation of the bronchial tree.

11. Correction of intracranial hypertension. To assess the critical limit of intracranial hypertension (ICH), CT examination of neurological status and objective monitoring based on dislocation symptoms should be performed and summarized. There are two ways to reduce HFH, the first is surgically - trepanation route. The second way is to reduce one of the components of the brain (blood, brain, and liquor).

HFH can occur due to the following causes: excessive motor excitation, fullness of the blood vessels of the brain, spasms, enlargement of inflamed and ischemic areas of the brain. Treatment of each of these causes should be individualized and treated with great care.

All sorts of combinations of different sedatives are used for this purpose:

- midozolam, a primary dose of 0.15 mg/kg, or diazepam 0.15 mg/kg+ ketamine together with a primary dose of 1.5 mg/kg of weight; and control doses should be administered by continuous infusion (every hour) in equal amounts.
- droperidol 0.15 mg/kg body weight in primary and regulatory doses+ ketamine 1.5 mg/kg body weight in primary and regulatory doses;
- Thiopental (5 mg/kg) or hexenal (7 mg/kg) weight+ ketamine 1.5 mg/kg weight in primary (bolus) and regulatory (every hour);
- sodium oxybutyrate (gamma - oxybutyric acid, GOSH) 50 mg/kg body weight+ midazolam (diazepam) 0.15 mg/kg body weight (every hour);
- promedolol 1 mg/kg weight in initial doses (bolus) and regulatory doses of 0.5 mg/kg/hour+ midazolam 0.15 mg/kg weight;
- fentanyl 5 mg/kg weight in both cases+ clofelin (administered by titration);
- propofol in initial doses (bolus) 2 mg/kg body weight, in regulatory doses (continuous infusion) 3 mg/kg body weight every hour.

Due to the fact that sedatives worsen the control of neurologic status and stuns cough reflexes, as well as, due to hemodynamic disturbances these drugs are used in limited amounts and with great caution.

12. Treatment and prevention of seizures. Drug treatment for early prevention of seizures has little effect. It is only when timely surgical intervention is performed that secondary brain damage can be prevented. It is very important that the therapeutic drugs used are administered intravenously and completely eliminate seizures. In order to eliminate such cases, it is important to point out two main useful points: - firstly, complete and rapid elimination of seizures gives good results.

- secondly, intravenous medication must be used to eliminate seizures. In case the desired effect is not achieved as a result, various combinations by means of a probe and parenteral administration are used, resulting in a prolonged effect with enteral administration and a rapid effect with parenteral administration.

To this end, diazepam 0.15-0.4 mg/kg body weight was administered at an infusion rate of 2.5 mg/minute or by drip at 0.1-0.2 mg/kg per hour. At the same time, the successful diazepam substitute midazolam 0.2-0.4 mg/kg and flunitrazepam (Rohypnol) 0.015-0.03 mg/kg as a replacement drug were used. The equivalence doses of the mentioned benzodiazepines were taken as follows: 1 mg flunitrazepam = 2 mg lorazepam =10 mg diazepam = 10 mg midazolam.

Valproic acid (Depakine) in the amount of 6 -7 mg / kg of weight intravenously for 3 - 5 minutes, four times a day is used as drugs of the 3rd line. Thiopental, being a component of the same series, is administered intravenously for 20 seconds in the amount of 250 - 300 mg, the subsequent rate is prescribed 5 - 8 mg / kg per hour.

Hexenal 6-8 mg/kg via bolus, brietal 1 - 3 mg/kg, and a regulatory dose of 2 - 4 mg/kg per hour were administered.

Sodium oxybutyrate and propofol are used in normal doses to provide controlled sedation and to eliminate seizures.

13. Neuroprotection. This concept means providing prevention of secondary brain complications, i.e. protecting neurons from damage (cytotoxins, ischemia, free radicals and others).

The main areas of neuroprotection are:

1) Control of hypercalcemia;

2) Reducing free radicals produced by "oxidative stress".

3) Use of excitatory amino acid antagonists (glutamate).

4) The use of drugs of neurotrophic influence.

5) Effects on glial cells and blockade of inflammatory responses;

6) Blockade and prevention of neuroglia and neuronal apoptosis.

In order to obtain a real effect from neuroprotection it is necessary to observe the following basic rules: intensive therapy must necessarily begin with ensuring adequate blood circulation and gas exchange. Neuroprotection should be initiated by providing adequate cerebral perfusion pressure from the first hours of injury and after gas exchange has been restored. To this end, the calcium antagonist Nimotop 10 mg twice daily was administered intravenously to combat secondary cerebral ischemia. For the purpose of free radical scavenging, intravenous "scavenging" antioxidants 10-30% vitamin E 1 ml 1 - 2 times a day were administered.

Of neuroprotectors with a wide range of effects, Glutatin 600 mg intravenously - intramuscularly 2 times a day was prescribed.

In cases of prevalent brain injury, Mexidol 1200 mg per day was prescribed.

Cortexin 20 mg per day was also prescribed.

14. Treatment of purulent-septic complications. For this purpose, along with the application of the method of A.P. Friedman, antibiotics and antiseptics were used from the first days of trauma.

For this purpose, to prevent meningitis, which are the main factors, a serious cleaning and sanitation of head and brain wounds was carried out. Among local antiseptics, 0.5-1% Dioxidine was applied intranasally, in the ear canal and in the oral cavity.

In order to prevent meningism, Chloramphenicol (levomycetin) parenterally 1 g every 12 hours was prescribed from antibiotics crossing the blood-brain barrier.

Once sensitivity has been established, various cephalosporins (3rd - 4th generation) are combined with antibacterial drugs. Combinations of meronem+ sultacin have been successfully used by us.

15. It is very important to regulate the activity of the organs damaged in different combinations of joint traumas, to prevent additional impulses from the shockogenic zones, to realize constant control of the damaged areas of the abdominal cavity organs.

For this purpose, blockades with 0.5% novocaine, 0.25% novocaine+ alcohol were performed in the cavities of the organs constituting the components of the community, and various medicinal and antiseptic dressings were applied.

16. Satisfaction of enteral nutrition and energy requirements. In order to eliminate the lack of plastic and energy materials as a result of hypercatabolism and hypermetabolism, as well as for the translocation of bacteria, it is necessary to carry out enteral nutrition.

For this purpose, enteral nutrition is carried out as early as possible by inserting a nasogastric tube. In order to ensure motor and evacuation functions, we used such ready-made nutritional preparations as Dipeptiven, Enjur and others, as well as amino acids and nutritional mixtures offered by us.

Aminoplasmol, which is a complex of amino acids, is administered intravenously by means of a probe 50 - 200 ml 3 times a day. After that, mixtures of milk+ sour cream+ honey + 1-2 pieces of uncooked eggs in the amount of 100 - 150 ml prepared at a certain temperature and in certain ratios are prescribed.

17. Nursing interventions. This package includes a wide range of physical, medication and even non-traditional care.

The following care measures, which we have implemented, are mandatory for the patients:

- The patient should be put to bed with the head elevated 30 degrees;
- Every 3 hours, the patient should be turned to a different position;
- 2 - 4 times a day you should clean your mouth and wipe your body;
- The bladder should be flushed 1-2 times a day with antiseptic;
- every other day it is necessary to make cleansing enemas from decoctions of sage or chamomile.

All the above requirements of the general treatment principles were followed and implemented for all patients (347 patients).

13. Principles of prevention and treatment of changes occurring in the gastroduodenal tract in combined severe craniocerebral trauma

In fractures of the skull base and facial skeleton in the aftermath of severe combined craniocerebral trauma, most of the blood drains into the gastric cavity. Filled into the stomach blood begins to break down under the influence of gastric acid and gastric juice, resulting in the formation of acidic hemotype compounds. It was found that the accumulation of more than 50 ml of blood in the stomach is accompanied by a gag reflex. Accumulation of blood in the stomach and sharp excitation by the products of cleavage of mucous membranes become the cause of gastric secretion with high acidity. At the same time, the products of blood cleavage lead to damage to the mucous gel, which performs barrier functions of the mucous membrane.

It can be said that in joint traumas vomiting syndromes, the sources of which are craniocerebral injuries and deep shock states, are observed in most cases. In severe brain injuries, intracranial hematomas, acute brain inflammation, vomiting syndromes are constantly observed and have indirect diagnostic value.

As a result of vomiting, bile and duodenal contents reflux into the stomach and esophagus. Bile acids entering the stomach begin to break down the mucoproteins of the mucosal barrier. The amount of gastric acid in the gastric contents increases, both in the gastric contents and in the blood. Along with the increase in the volume of gastritis, there is an increase in the volume of histamine in the blood, resulting in increased sensitization, due to which local allergic antibody reactions occur in the mucous membranes and mucosal layer. As a result of local microcirculatory disorders and immune system insufficiency, pathological changes in the mucous membranes further deepen and at later stages turn into erosions and ulcers.

Hypovolemic and hypoxic conditions of various degrees, exacerbation of inflammatory processes, the emergence of infection in the process of damage, abnormalities occurring in the hemostasis system, further deepen pathological changes in the mucous membranes. In order to prevent the transition to erosions and ulcers pathological changes occurring in the mucous membranes of the gastroduodenum under the influence of acute and sharp stress factors as a result of injuries, an important and urgent problem is the implementation of early preventive and therapeutic measures.

Measures taken for this purpose shall include the following principles:

1) Removal of accumulated blood and bile acids in the stomach by gastric probing, gastric lavage, gastric decompression, enteral administration of drugs to patients deprived of the swallowing act, and implementation of comprehensive measures to nourish the patient;

2) Implementation of therapeutic measures to improve local blood supply and microcirculation;

3) Implementation of therapeutic measures to enhance regeneration and repair processes in the mucous membranes of the gastroduodenum;

4) Implementation of therapeutic measures aimed at strengthening the immune system in the mucous membranes of the gastro-duodenum;

5) Implementation of therapeutic measures that provide regulation of motor - evacuation functions and regulation of gastric pH.

6) Implementation of therapeutic measures aimed at preventing the development of Helikobacter pilori in the gastro-duodenal environment;

- In the early stages, the stomach is decompressed by probing, the blood and masses of food filled in the stomach are cleared. Periodic gastric lavage with clean water is performed. Corrective measures are implemented for changes assessed by endoscopic and pH-metric examinations. By means of a probe, coagulating antocidal drugs (Almagel, Maalox, etc.) are administered. In cases where there is a possibility of enteral nutrition, nutrition is carried out by probing, at the same time creating conditions for the determination of bile acids and sialic acids in the stomach contents. Along with the therapeutic and diagnostic value of probing there are other effects. Thus, after prolonged probing processes in the esophagus and gastric mucous membranes, mechanical injuries and wounds may occur.

- Therapeutic measures to improve microcirculation are carried out on general and local principles. The complex of general measures includes therapeutic measures directed against shock situations, improvement of rheological features of blood, elimination of hypovolemia and hypoxia, anti-inflammatory and anti-infectious measures. As local treatment measures are used brews of sea buckthorn oil, vinylin solution (Shostakovsky's balsam), other mixed brews.

- In order to increase the regenerative ability of mucous membranes individually prescribed dalargin, actovegin, solcoseryl.

- In order to strengthen the immune capacity of the mucous membranes inside prescribed syrup peritol, glutatin solution (dipeptiven).

- Along with cleansing enemas to purify the pH of the stomach and restore the motor - evacuation functions, and along with gastric lavage with cold water simultaneously with a solution of 25% - g magnesium sulfate 20 - 30 ml of cholinomimetics used Proserin or Ubrethit.

- In order to prevent the development of Helicobacterpilori in the stomach, Metranidazole or Secnidox is administered orally.

The principles of measures taken to prevent the transition into erosions and ulcers of pathological changes occurring in the mucous membranes of the gastroduodenum under the influence of acute and sharp stress factors as a result of trauma are summarized in the following table (Table 5.1).

14. Principles of prevention and treatment of pathologic changes occurring in the mucous membranes of gastroduodenum and duodenum

Table 5.1.

Principles of the package of measures	Therapeutic methods used
Decompression, protection *and* cleansing	Gastric probing, cold water lavage, initiation of early enteral nutrition (full or passive).
Improvement of microcirculation and local blood supply	Reopolyglukin, actovegin, curantil, trental intravenously, sea buckthorn oil, vinylin solution inside.
Improvement of regenerative and reparative processes of mucous membranes	Intramuscular dalargin, plasmol.
Improving the immune capacity of mucous membranes	Peritol syrup, glutamine solution (dipeptivin), immunoglobulin 25 ml intravenously, thymolin, T - activin intramuscularly.
Regulation of pH and motor and evacuation functions of the stomach	Inside or intramuscularly almagel, zantac, kvamatel. Intravenously 20 - 30 ml of magnesium sulphate. Intramuscularly with proserine, cerucal or ubretide.
Helicobacter pilori prevention	Metranidazole orally.

Along with the implemented therapeutic measures is very important to implement from the first day of injury full or partial enteral nutrition of patients. At this time, it is necessary to ensure that there is no aspiration of food into the bronchi and no retention of contents in the gastric tube.

The complex of therapeutic measures was realized on 347 patients of the main group, subjected to traditional therapeutic measures and on 200 patients from this group, to whom measures aimed at regulation of vagoinsular-enteric systems were applied. The implemented therapeutic measures gave the following results:

- 246 patients (70.9%) recovered,
- 91 patients (26.2%) had a fatal outcome.

From the main indicators. Characterizing the clinical condition of patients, regulation of motor - evacuation functions of the gastro-duodenum, elimination of aggressive influences of gastric pH and bile acids in the stomach and the results of the influence of retained contents were evaluated on the basis of endoscopic parameters.

The effectiveness of therapeutic measures in deep inflammatory processes in the mucous membrane of the gastro-duodenal intestine, and in reducing the incidence of acute erosions and ulcers and their accompaniment by acute bleeding were taken as the main parameters to be evaluated.

Acute erosions and ulcers were found in 31 patients (21.1%) out of 147 in the main group who were treated with conventional therapeutic measures, of which 14 patients (9.5%) had bleeding complications.

Twenty-three (11.5%) of the 200 patients in the main group who were treated with measures aimed at regulating the vagoinsular-enteric system were found to have acute erosions and ulcers, of which 7 patients (3.5%) had bleeding complications.

Based on endoscopic examinations, it was found that acute erosions and ulcers occurred most frequently on the 3rd - 5th day of trauma, and on the 5th - 7th day damage to the abdominal, thoracic, and pulmonary organs and were most common in these combinations of compatibility.

The partial superficiality of inflammatory processes, superficial and sporadic nature of the detected erosions and ulcers attracted attention as the main indicators of the effectiveness of preventive and therapeutic measures.

15. Principles of regulation of changes in peptides of vagoinsular and enteric systems in patients of the main group with combined craniocerebral trauma

In response to disturbances occurring in the metabolic system to adaptive reactions of the adreno-cortical system against acute stress factors as a result of synergistic activity of the vagoinsular and enteric systems, processes of hypercatabolism and hypermetabolism occur. Damage to hypothalamic-pituitary structures plays a major role in the development of these processes. As a result of the acceleration of the breakdown of transverse striated muscles, the loss of nitrogen in the urine increases. Excessive increase in catabolism leads to immune disorders and reduction of other vital proteins - albumin and globulin due to disturbances in the processes of antibody secretion in the synthesis of active substances.

Hyperglycemia is another common form of metabolic abnormalities. During severe joint trauma, hyperglycemia leads to prognosis with severe neurologic outcomes. Thus, hypoxia and hyperglycemia cause the development of lacto acidosis. In addition, during hyperglycemia, some glucose is converted to excitotoxic amino acids.

Despite the increase in insulin secretion as a result of early vagoinsular influences, less insulin is found outside the portal system than is actually synthesized. The major part of insulin (90%), which has a universal anabolic influence, passing through the blood vessels on the background of hyperglycemia, is utilized in the blood system of the liver. During the conversion of inactive proinsulin into insulin, C-peptide is released, consisting of 23- x amino acid residues, which cannot carry hormonal functions and does not have highly sensitive receptors like insulin. Therefore, an increase in the volume of C-peptide outside the portal system during high blood cortisol concentrations is evaluated as an indirect indicator of increased insulin secretion and is considered one of the signs of insulin resistance.

Along with the increase in insulin secretion, highly acidic gastric juice is secreted, which becomes the cause of increased gastritis.

Enteric peptides passing into the blood enter into communication with cells of the mucous layer and become the cause of histamine release. And histamine, in its turn, increases membrane permeability of mucous membrane cells and creates conditions for even more intensification of secretion and influx of regulatory peptides into the blood.

Thus, regulation of the activity of the vagoinsular and enteric systems, which complement each other and are in interrelation with each other, is one of the topical issues.

For this purpose, it is recommended to apply to patients from the moment of admission native plasma and erythrocyte mass of the same group in accordance with the volume of blood lost.

Inhalation of $O_2\uparrow$ or an artificial breathing regimen enriched with $O_{(2)\uparrow}$ is necessary to eliminate hypoxia.

In order to eliminate the effects exerted on metabolic processes by vagoinsular peptides, patients are intravenously administered Trisol simultaneously with administration of solutions Ringer+ Sodium bicarbonate 8.4% + Riboxin and of antioxidants Mexidol 5 ml 2 times a day, Vitamin E 30% - 1 ml. In order to regulate these peptides at subsequent stages and to correct hyperglycemia, patients are administered 6-10 units of insulin subcutaneously, or as polarized mixtures intravenously (NaCl 0.9%- 300 ml+ panangin 10 ml+ cocarboxylase 100 mg+ Novocain 0.5%- 200 ml+ insulin 6-10 units).

For enzymatic regulation of metabolism the patients were prescribed Wobenzyme 1 tablet x 3 times a day by dissolving in water and administered by nasogastric tube.

Taking into account the increased concentration of gastritis, under the influence of high acid secretion in order to regulate enteric peptides, the stomachs of the patients were flushed with alkaline waters of 12-15 C, after which enteral nutrition was carried out earlier and of the antacid preparations one (Almagel, Maalox, etc.) was prescribed intravenously 3 times a day. In cases where persistently high pH was observed in the evenings, H_2-blockers (Zantac or Simethidine intramuscularly, Quamatel intravenously) were administered intravenously or intramuscularly. H_2-blockers were used in limited quantities, given the conditions for the development of respiratory tract infections.

Suprastin or Tavegil 1 ml x 2 times intravenously or intramuscularly were administered to regulate the increase in histamine and to eliminate side effects (Arthus phenomenon in the gastric mucosa).

Sandostatin 50 - 100 mg intravenously 2 times daily for 5 -7 days was prescribed to regulate Samostatin.

Therapeutic measures aimed at regulating vagoinsular and enteric peptides were implemented on 200 patients. Depending on the combinations of compatibility, the number of patients was as follows:

- with severe craniocerebral trauma accompanied by combined fractures of bones of legs and pelvis - 67 people;

- with severe craniocerebral - brain trauma accompanied by combined injuries of abdominal cavity organs - 82 people;

- with severe craniocerebral - brain trauma accompanied by combined injuries of the chest, ribs and lungs - 51 people.

Along with the therapeutic measures aimed at regulation of vagoinsular and enteric systems in the main group, all the requirements of the general principles of the applied treatment were implemented in the patients of the general group.

Out of the whole group, 51 patients (25.5%) were noted to be fatal. Of these:

- 21 patients (10.5%) - on the 1-2nd day;
- 17 patients (8.5%) - on the 5th-7th day;
- 13 patients (6.5%) - on the 7-9th day after traumatization.

The cause of death in 39 patients (19.5%) was acute brain tumor as a consequence of severe brain damage and intracerebral hematomas.

In 12 patients (6%) the cause of death was determined to be organ and system insufficiency according to combinations of compatibility against the background of severe craniocerebral traumas.

Of the 200 patients who received therapeutic measures aimed at regulating the vagoinsular and enteric systems, 7 patients (3.5%) had acute erosions and ulcers in the gastroduodenal system complicated by bleeding.

Fibrogastroscopic examination performed on patients in whom bleeding complications were noted revealed as sources of bleeding:

- acute erosion in 5 patients and combination of acute erosion and ulcers in 2 patients.
- In 2 out of 5 patients erosions were found in the duodenum, and in 5 patients - in the cardiac part and on the small curvature of the stomach.
- In 2 x patients, acute erosions were noted in the cardiac part and small curvature of the stomach, as well as in the bulb of the duodenum.

In 149 people (74.5%) the treatment was completed with recovery. Taking into account that the main component of compatibility is craniocerebral injuries, constant attention was paid to the period of comatose state of patients and assessment of their neurological status.

According to the combinations of compatibility, the period of duration of coma of the patients was as follows:

- with severe craniocerebral trauma accompanied by combined fractures of leg and pelvis bones: in 17 patients (25.3%) on the 1st day, in 31 patients (46.3%) on the 2nd day, in 19 patients (28.3%) on the 3rd day.
- with severe craniocerebral trauma accompanied by combined injuries of abdominal cavity organs: in 32 patients (39.02%) 1 day, in 29 patients (35.4%) 3 days, in 21 patients (25.6%) 5 days;
- with severe craniocerebral trauma accompanied by combined injuries of the thorax, ribs and

lungs: in 17 patients (33.3%) 1 day, in 23 patients (45.1%) 3 days, in 11 patients (21.5%) 5 days.

Results of therapeutic interventions aimed at regulating the vagoinsular and enteric systems:

- Regulation of vagoinsular peptide values and maintenance within the normal range;
- Regulation of enteric peptide values and maintenance within the normal range;
- In addition, the results were evaluated based on a set of measures of organ and system regulation and other parameters, and aimed at meeting the needs of traditional treatment and the objectives of this study.

The detection of bleeding complications of acute erosions and ulcers in 33 patients (9.5%) out of 347 patients in the patient group, in 14 patients (9.5%) out of 147 patients receiving conventional treatment, and in 7 patients (3.5%) out of 200 patients treated with therapeutic measures aimed at regulating the vagoinsular and enteric systems, was evaluated as parameters of treatment outcome. While in the observed group 33 patients had complications accompanied by bleeding, in the same number of patients from the main group (347 patients) only 21 patients (6.1%) had such complications. The main part of bleeding complications was found in patients with craniocerebral trauma accompanied by combined injuries of abdominal cavity organs (4 patients) and in patients with craniocerebral trauma accompanied by combined injuries of chest and lung organs (3 patients).

Reduction in the incidence of complications of acute erosions and bleeding ulcers was evaluated as the main parameters of treatment indicators.

In order to eliminate hyperglycemia it is necessary to inject patients subcutaneously 6 - 10 units of insulin, or in the form of polarized mixtures intravenously (NaCl 0.9%-300 ml+ panangin 10 ml+ cocarboxylase 100 mg+ Novocain 0.5%- 200 ml+ insulin 6-10 units).

In order to eliminate the effects of highly acidic gastric secretions, the stomachs of patients should be flushed with cold water, after which one of the antacid preparations should be administered into the stomach cavity. In cases of persistently high pH in the evenings, intravenous or intramuscular administration of H_2-blockers (Zantac or Simethidine intramuscularly, Quamatel intravenously) is recommended.

Suprastin or Tavegil intravenously or intramuscularly is administered to regulate the increase in histamine and eliminate side effects (Arthus phenomenon in the gastric mucosa).

16. Tactics and principles of treatment of complications with gastric bleeding

In the formation of acute erosions and ulcers under the influence of vagoinsular and enteral mechanisms during severe craniocerebral trauma as a result of the constant influence of these factors and other pathogenetic mechanisms in the subsequent stages of the disease can occur complications with bleeding in correlation with disorders of hemostasis.

Depending on the amount of blood loss during bleeding complications, manifested by various clinical signs (hypotension, collaptoid states, cold sweats, melena, brownish sludge, etc.), melena of various degrees and vomiting with brownish sludge (discharge of brownish sludge or blood from the gastric tube) usually attract attention in the early period.

After gastric lavage with cold water until the stomach is completely cleansed, fibrogastroduodenoscopy is performed. As a result of this manipulation, which has both diagnostic and therapeutic value, there is detailed information about the location and nature of acute erosions and ulcers, as well as taking biopsy specimens for examination.

In case of detection of ongoing bleeding during endoscopic examinations, increased risk of erosions and bleeding ulcers (in the case of large diameter veins), local coagulation of ulcers and nearby areas (aminocarponic acid + 2% novocaine) with the use of biological adhesives (statisol, gastrozol) is performed.

Taking into account central hemodynamics, microcirculation, transcapillary exchange. Oxygen metabolism, acute disorders of defense reactions. Depending on the degree of blood loss, the correct implementation of transfusion treatment is important.

We have conditionally divided blood loss into three degrees:

1) Blood loss up to 25% is mild;

2) Blood loss of up to 30-40% is severe;

3) Blood loss of up to 40% or more is massive blood loss.

During bleeding events, blood transfusion operations should be performed based on serious indications.

During mild blood loss, the transfusion volume is recommended in the following composition: colloids 0.6 liters, crystalloids 1.0 liter (total 1.6 liters); during severe blood loss: colloids 1.0 - 1.5 liters, crystalloids 1.5 - 2.01 liters (total 3.3-4.7 liters); in massive blood loss: colloids 1.5 - 2.0 liters, crystalloids 2.0 - 2.5 liters (total 4.2-5.2 liters).

In severe blood loss, hemotransfusion should be 0.8-1.2 liters, and in massive blood loss - from 1.2

liters, and should be carried out at the expense of erythrocyte mass and fresh frozen plasma.

Despite the implementation of local and general hemostatic therapeutic measures, the finding of 60% to 70% blood loss should be taken as an indication for surgical intervention.

Treatment measures for bleeding complications are summarized in the following table: (Table 5.2).

Principles of treatment for bleeding complications

Table 5.2.

Components of topical, infusion and transfusion treatment administered	**Degrees of blood loss**		
	Weak (25%)	**Strong (30-40%)**	**Massive (40% ≥)**
General hemostatic treatment	+	+	+
Local endoscopic coagulation	+	+	+
An intravenous "noradrenaline test"	+	+	+
Ratio of crystalloids to colloids	1: 1	2: 1	3: 2
Erythrocyte mass	-	0,8-1,2 l	≥ 1,2 l
Native plasma	+	+	+
Drugs that improve local regeneration	+	+	+
Antacids and H_2-blockers	+	+	+

The common hemostatic treatment measures included: Dicinone intravenously and intramuscularly, Aminocaproic acid intravenously, Transamin-E intramuscularly, Calcium chlorine 10% intravenously, native plasma intravenously.

Local endoscopic coagulation measures consist of performing coagulation of erosions and ulcers and using biological adhesives.

Oral administration of hemostatic "noradrenaline test" is performed after flushing with cold water or aminocaproic acid by administering orally in cold water every 15 minutes on the first day and 3 times a day on the following days (4 ml noradrenaline+ adroxan 3 ml+ thrombin 300 mg+ aminocaproic acid 5% - 200 ml+ physiologic solution 300 ml). Ethoxysclerol is administered topically.

Colloids and crystalloids should be administered in a strictly observed ratio, intracellular and extracellular fluid deficiency should not be allowed.

Hemotransfusion should ensure that hemoglobin is maintained above 70% and the normal level of oxygen supply to brain tissue. In severe cases, 750 ml of red cell mass may be administered simultaneously. In such cases, attention should be paid to complications that may occur in the lungs.

In order to improve the processes of regeneration of acute erosions and ulcers recommended: Solcoseril - Actovegin intravenously and intramuscularly: Dalargin intramuscularly; Sea Buckthorn oil and Vinyl solution internally.

From antacid drugs and H_2 - blockers - Almagel, barium sulfate orally, Cimetidine, Ranitidine,

Famotidine, Zantac are prescribed in the evenings intravenously or intramuscularly.

17. Step-by-step principles of treatment of patients from the main group

The step-by-step principles of treatment of 347 patients from the main group of people with severe craniocerebral injuries were realized by dividing the patients into two groups. Traditional methods of treatment were applied to 147 patients. This set of measures, combining the general principles of treatment, was implemented on the following number of patients according to the combinations of injury compatibility. The number of patients to whom traditional methods of treatment were applied and the combinations of craniocerebral trauma compatibility were as follows:

1. with severe craniocerebral trauma accompanied by combined fractures of leg and pelvic bones - 43 people;
2. with severe craniocerebral trauma accompanied by combined injuries of abdominal cavity organs - 61 people;
3. with severe craniocerebral trauma accompanied by combined injuries of the chest, ribs and lungs - 53 people.

As already mentioned, all points and requirements of the general principles of treatment were realized. Of these, the lethal outcome of 40 patients (27%) was noted. The death of these patients occurred:

- 17 people - on the 1st - 3rd day of the disease;
- 13 people - on the 5th - 9th day of the disease;
- 10 people - on the 9th day of the disease.

The cause of death in 38 patients was cerebral and various systems disorders, in 2 patients - acute erosions and ulcers with complication of bleeding - profuse bleeding in the gastrointestinal system on the background of these disorders.

Bleeding complications of acute erosions and ulcers were noted in 14 (9.5%) patients out of 147 patients receiving conventional treatment.

In patients with bleeding complications of acute erosions and ulcers, the sources of bleeding were identified during endoscopic examinations:

- 4 patients had multiple acute erosions in different regions of the stomach;
- 2 patients had acute duodenal erosions;
- 2 patients had acute ulcers in the antral part and small curvature of the stomach;
- 2 patients had acute duodenal ulcers;

- 2 patients had acute ulcers simultaneously in the stomach and duodenum;
- 2 patients had exacerbation of chronic duodenal ulcers.

In 107 individuals (72.8%), treatment resulted in recovery.

Taking into account that the main component of compatibility is craniocerebral injuries, constant attention was paid to the period of coma of the patients and assessment of their neurological status.

According to the combinations of compatibility, the period of duration of coma of the patients was as follows:

- with severe craniocerebral trauma accompanied by combined fractures of leg and pelvis bones: in 13 patients (24.5%) on the 1st day, in 21 patients (39.6%) on the 2nd day, in 19 patients (35.8%) on the 3rd day.
- with severe craniocerebral trauma accompanied by joint injuries of abdominal cavity organs: in 21 patients (34.4%) 3 days, in 27 patients (44.3%) 5 days, in 13 patients (21.3%) 7 days;
- with severe craniocerebral trauma accompanied by combined injuries of the thorax, ribs and lungs: in 11 patients (33.3%) 3 days, in 15 patients (45.4%) 5 days, in 7 patients (21.2%) 7 days.

200 patients from the main group in addition to the traditional treatment measures were applied the therapeutic measures developed by us and at the early stages by means of a probe, and at the subsequent stages per os orally was administered a mixture made by us (bloodwort+ yarrow+ nettle roots; in the ratio 4:3:2:1) to purify the peptides of the vagoinsular and enteric systems and to provide protection of the mucous membranes of the gastric-duodenal intestinal system.

A set of the above measures was applied below to a specified number of patients based on compatibility combinations:

1. with severe craniocerebral trauma accompanied by combined fractures of leg and pelvic bones - 50 patients;
2. with severe craniocerebral trauma accompanied by combined injuries of abdominal cavity organs - 75 patients;
3. with severe craniocerebral trauma accompanied by combined injuries of the thorax, ribs and lungs - 75 patients.

The general principles of treatment (traditional) of patients from this group were applied along with the application of all the principles of treatment complexes developed by us.

The lethal outcome of the patients occurred:

- 15 people for 1-3- and a day

- 12 people on the 5th-9th day
- 9 people on the 9th day after injury.

The cause of death in 36 patients was disorders in the brain and other various systems (brain tumor, malignant hyperthermia, destructive processes in the lungs, pulmonary-cardiac insufficiency with a centralized source).

Complications of acute erosions and ulcers of the gastro-duodenal intestinal system with bleeding were noted in 7 patients. Of them 6 patients had gastric tube discharge with brownish sediment and short-term melena. And in one patient blood was discharged from the gastric tube along with the contents, and the intensity of melena was noted.

In patients with bleeding complications of acute erosions and ulcers, the sources of bleeding were identified during endoscopic examinations:

- 6 patients had erythromatous gastrobulbitis accompanied by point erosions of antral part;
- 1 patient had reflex esophagitis, erythromatous gastrobulbitis accompanied by numerous pitting erosions of the antral part and duodenum.

Clinical observation:

Patient: X

Age: 31

Medical history: #2709

Diagnosis: combined craniocerebral trauma, brain damage. Fracture of both femurs, right shoulder and right sciatic bone.

On KT examination: hemorrhagic foci in the left internal capsule, cortical areas of hemorrhage were found in the left parietal lobe and forehead, and there were residuals in the paranasal sinuses.

On the 14th day of treatment, 48 hours after nutritive feeding of the patient, there was a discharge from the gastric tube, first with brownish residue and then with blood. Also, melena was noted in the patient.

Results of esophagogastroduodenoscopy: reflux esophagitis. Erythematous gastrobulbitis accompanied by pinpoint erosions of the antral part. After complex conservative treatment measures the bleeding was stopped, no recurrence was noted.

155 (77.5%) of the 200 patients in the main group who received comprehensive treatment measures showed recovery, while the remaining 45 (22.5%) cases were fatal. The timing of coma was traced as follows depending on the combinations of compatibility:

- with severe craniocerebral trauma accompanied by combined fractures of leg and pelvis bones: in 30 patients (60%) 1 day, in 14 patients (28%) 2 days, in 6 patients (12%) 3 days.

- with severe craniocerebral trauma accompanied by combined injuries of abdominal cavity organs: in 13 patients (17.3%) 3 days, in 33 patients (44%) 5 days, in 9 patients (12%) 7 days;

- with severe craniocerebral trauma accompanied by combined injuries of the thorax, ribs and lungs: in 40 patients (53.3%) 3 days, in 20 patients (26.7%) 5 days, in 15 patients (20%) 7 days.

Along with the regulation of vagoinsular and enteric system peptides, in the main group of patients who were treated with the complex of therapeutic and prophylactic measures developed by us, the dynamics of examined peptides, pH of gastric contents, bile acids in the stomach and free sialic acids indices was as follows (Table 5.9.1).

Table 5.9.1.

Dynamics of the examined parameters in patients of the main group who regulation of vagoinsular and enteric systems (200 patients).

Indicators to be checked	**Days of surveys**							
	I	**III**	**V**	**VII**	**IX**	**XII**	**XV**	**XVIII**
Insulin μmv / ml	21,08± 0,71**	20,11± 0,57*	11,09± 0,55	9,19± 0,41	8,13±0 ,33	7,18±0 ,27	7,09±0 ,17	6,31±0 ,11
C - peptide ng / ml	4,09±0, 16	3,71±0 ,13	3,51±0 ,9	2.33± 0.7	2,27±0 ,7	2,21±0 ,3	2,13±0 ,4	2,11±0 ,3
Gastrin pg/mL	121,33 ±2,51	109,21 ±1,03	88,11± 0,15	76,31 ±0,11	71,27± 0,9	67,13± 0,3	63,11± 0,1	61,17± 0,1
Histamine mcg, %	12,9±0, 4	11,7+0 ,3	11,1±0 ,3	9,3±0, 4	8,3±0, 2	7,5±0, 1	6,1±0,3	5,3±0, 1
stomach pH	4,06±0, 13	3,74±0 ,11	3,63±0 ,09	3,31± 0,21	3,17±0 ,13	3,11±0 ,11	3,11±0 ,05	3,09±0 ,09
Bile acids in stomach mg / l	0,61±0, 03	0,21±0 ,03	0,12±0 ,02	0,7±0, 02	0,6±0, 01	0,17±0 ,02	0,13±0 ,01	0,11±0 ,01
Free sialic acid in stomach μmol/L	23,3±0, 9	21,1±1 ,3	20,5±0 ,3	19,1± 0,3	18,1±0 ,1	19,3±0 ,3	18,1±0 ,1	17,3±0 ,3

As can be seen from the table, in spite of the fact that the examined indices on the first day were observed at high doses, at the subsequent stages it turned out to be possible to maintain them within the normal range.

Results of the treatment performed:

- regulation of motor - evacuation functions of the gastro-duodenal intestinal system;
- elimination of residual substances from the stomach contents;
- Minimizing the concentration of bile acids and free sialic acid in gastric contents.
- Maintaining the pH of the stomach within normal limits;

- maintaining normal blood sugar and saturation (SPO_2) levels in peripheral blood.
- Ensuring the daily energy requirement, regulation of nutritive nutrition and electrolyte balance;
- early prevention of infections and inflammatory processes and regulation of other parameters.

18. Schematic mechanisms of occurrence of acute erosions and ulcers

Scheme 1

Shock and coma due to severe trauma	Increase in adaptation hormones, increase in catobolism
Blood loss, centralization of blood circulation due to shocks and disturbances in the activity of the central system Microcirculatory disturbances	
Effect of the vagoinsular system on the insular apparatus, increasing insulin release	Microcirculatory disorders in the mucous membranes of the gastroduodenal - 12-intestinal system
Increased activity of the enteric system, increased concentrations of gastrin and histamine	Reflux of bile into the stomach, the destructive effect of the breakdown products of blood and bile acids filled into the stomach on the mucosal barrier of the stomach
Appearance of small necrotic foci in mucous membranes, signs of Arthus phenomenon of local inflammation.	
Continuation of disorders of motor - evacuation activity of the gastric - 12-typer intestinal system	Continued reflux of bile into the stomach on the background of microcirculatory disorders
Continued disturbance of the acid-alkaline balance of the stomach contents	Destruction by bile acids of the protective functions of the mucosal barrier, increase in the amount of free sialic acid in gastric contents
Formation of acute erosions and ulcers based on the noted polyetiologic and pathogenetic mechanisms	
Weakening of the immune system against the background of increased catabolism, pathologic effect of pancreatic hormones on venous permeability, increased thyroid hormones (T_3, T_4)	Increased immune lysis reactions during the development of inflammatory changes and infections
Deepening of acute erosions and ulcers in the gastroduodenal and 12-intestinal system	Increased immuno - lysis reactions, hyperthermia, a - Amylase, impaired fibrinolytic system
Complication of acute erosions and ulcers, formed against the background of the noted pathogenetic mechanisms, under the influence of disorders of the fibrinolytic system	

19. Markers of vagoinsular and enteric systems in the formation of acute erosions and ulcers

In the blood:

- cortisol;
- e-peptide;
- glucohemoglobin;
- somatostatin;
- insulin;
- gastrin;
- sialic acid;
- E-reactive protein;
- antistreptolysin;
- hemoglobin, platelets, fibrinogen, prothrombin index

In the stomach contents:

- pH adjustment
- bile acid determination
- Establishment of free, bound and weakly bound sialic acids
- Helicobacter pilori.

In groups in which elevated levels of these indicators were observed, the formation of acute erosions and ulcers in the mucous membranes of the gastro-duodenal intestinal system was found. The increased level of these indicators in patients with complications in the form of bleeding attracts attention.

20. REFERENCE LIST

1. Hasanov R.S., Etibarli S.A Neurosurgery. Baku, 2004, pp. 123131

2. Isaev H.B.. Pathophysiology of surgical diseases. Baku, "Nurlan" printed edition, 2005, pp.26-31

3. Ismailov I.S. "Resuscitation: principles, stages and methods". Textbook. Baku. 2007. 174 pp.

4. Guliyev Ch.B. Craniocerebral traumas in children. Baku, printed edition of AMU, 2007, pp.55-58.

5. Guliyev Ch.B.Children's traumatology. AMU Press, Baku, 2004, pp. 21-38.

6. Yusifov A.A. Peculiarities of treatment and prevention of brain edema in craniocerebral traumas. Chemistry, Biology, Medical Journal, 2002,№ 1, pp.82-84.

7. Alkim H, Şaşmaz N. Akut üst gastrointestinal sistem kanaması. Ozden A, Şahin B,Yılmaz U, Soykan İ (ed). Gastroenteroloji. 1. baski. Ankara: Fersa Matbaacilik; 2002. 141-148.

8. Boyükuncu Y. Üst gastrointestinal sistem endoskopisi. Kalayci G (ed). Genel Cerrahi. 1.baski. İstanbul: Nobel Tip Kitab evleri; 2002. Cilt 2: 10291049.

9. Gokşen Y. Peptik ülser ve stress gastriti. Kalayci G (ed). Genel Cerrahi. 1. baskı. Istanbul: Nobel Tip Kitab evleri; 2002. Cilt 2: 973-1003.

10. Gürel S, Imadoglu O. Varis ve malignite dişi üst gastrointestinal system kanamalarinin degerlendirilmesi. Uludag üniversitesi Tip Fakültesi Dergisi 2004;2:87-91.

11. Kayaçetin E., Polat H. Üst gastrointestinal sistem kanamalari: 52 vakanin incelenmesi. Genel Tip Dergisi 2003; 13: 119-122.

12. Küçükardali Y, Yazgan Y. Geriatrik populasyonda nonsteroidal antiinflamatuar ilaçlara bagli olan ve olmayan üst gastrointestinal sistem kanamali olgularin karşilaştirilmasi. Turkish Journal of Geriatrics 2002, 5:87-90.

13. Ozmen V, Avci C, Avtan L. Videoendoskopik gastrik cerrahi. Avci C, Avtan L (ed). Videoskopik Cerrahi. 1. baski. Istanbul: Avrupa Tip Kitapsilik; 2000. 316-331.

14. Memik F. Peptik ülser komplikasionlari. In: Memik F (ed). Her Yonüyle Peptik Ülser. Istanbul: Nobel tip Kitap evleri, 2003: 105-112.

15. Memisoglu K. Akut üst gastrointestinal sistem kanamalari. Türkiye Klinikleri J Surg Med Sci. 2005; 1(4):1-6

16. Paksoy M, Yavuz N. Akut üst gastrointestinal sistem kanamasinda mortaliteyi etkileyen risk

faktorleri. T klin Surgery 2000;5:53-8.

17. Polat Y., Celebi F. Hemostaz, carrahi kanamalar va kontransfuzionu. Genel cerrahi. Istanbul, 2002, s. 95-108

18. Saribeyoglu K. Mide. Ergüney S, Çiçek Y (Çeviri ed). Güncel Cerrahi Tedavi. 6. baski. Istanbul: Avrupa Tip Kitapsilik; 2001. Cilt 1 : 77-122.

19. Sonmez MF, Ozan E. Açlik ve açlik sonrasi doyurulmanin siçan mide dokusu üzerine etkileri: φik mikroskobik çalφma. Firat Tip Dergisi 2005; 10: 96-102.

20. Silverstein FE, Faich G, Goldsiein JL: Osteoartrit ve romatoid artritte kullanilan selekoksib ve NSAiPlarin gastrointestinal toksisite açisindan karşilaştirilmasi. JAMA 2000:284: 1247-1255.

21. Torüner M. Gastrointestinal hastaliklarm belirtileri. Geçim Ì E (çeviri ed). Cerrahinin Ìlkeleri. 1. baski. Ankara: Antip; 2004. 1053-1100.

22. Türel O. Gastrointestinal kanamalar. Kalayci G (ed). Genel Cerrahi. 1. baski. Ìstanbul: Nobel Tip Kitabevleri; 2002. Cilt 1: 271-282.

23. Aleksandrov B.H., Bobriyskaya I.G., Karmolina L.F. Syndrome of disseminated intravascular blood coagulation and its significance in craniocerebral trauma / Mosk. med. stomatol. inst. named after N.A. Semashko. N.A. Semashko. Moscow, 2002, 49p. - dep. B UNMB

24. Ammar H.A. Choice of surgeon's tactics in bleeding from acute erosive-ulcerous lesions of the stomach and duodenum: Cand. of Medical Sciences. St. Petersburg, 2001. - 22 c.

25. Ankin L.N. "Polytrauma (organizational, tactical and methodological problems). Moscow. Med.press-inform., 2004, 176 p.

26. Artemiev E.V., Korshakova I.V. Clinic and treatment of combined craniocerebral trauma accompanied by shock / Combined trauma and traumatic shock. Respubl. sb. of scientific works. Moscow, 2001, pp. 56-63.

27. Astrakov C. B. Possibilities of antioxidant therapy in limiting secondary brain damage in neuroresuscitation patients // Bulletin of Experimental Biology and Medicine, 2006, appendix 1, p. 176.

28. Asfarammeshginshahr Sadegh. Possibilities of conservative hemostasis in acute gastroduodenal ulcer bleeding: Cand. of Medicine. Mosk. med. akad. - Moscow, 2005 - 24 p.

29. Balatanova E.D., Volny I.F. Pomerantseva T.I. et al. "Intensive therapy of critical conditions at the prehospital stage". Lugansk: Shiko, 2009, 120 p.

30. Berdiev R.N. Craniocerebral trauma with severe clinical course // Bulletin of Surgery, 2005,№

6, p.97. -100

31. Bokeria L.A., Yarustovsky M.B., Shipova E.A. Acute gastroduodenal bleeding in cardiovascular surgery. - M., 2004. - 186 c.

32. Borodulina E.V. Vegetative dysregulation in gastric ulcer and duodenal ulcer and its correction by synaptotropic preparations: Author's abstract. 2003, Tomsk. -48 c.

33. A.F. Buzunov Formation of psychosomatic pathology. Ulcer disease. Gallstone disease.

34. Vakhidov A.V., Muradov M.K.. External respiratory function and pulmonary hemodynamics in patients with neurotrauma // Voprosy neurosurgery named after Acad. N.N. Burdenko, 2001,№ 3, pp. 16-19.

35. Vvedensky V.P., Zabusov A.V., Zhbannikov P.S. Opportunities of bronchoscopy in the diagnosis and treatment of aspiration in victims with severe craniocerebral trauma // Intensive Care Bulletin, 2005,№ 2, p.66.

36. Vedernikov .E. Clinical and pathogenetic characterization of chronic (complete) gastroduodenal erosions and their differentiated treatment: Cand. of medical sciences.-Perm, 2000.-105 p.

37. Vereshchagin E.I., Vereshchagin I.P. "Intensive therapy of severe and combined craniocerebral trauma". Novosibirsk. 2007. 85 c.

38. Vinnik Y.S., Kartel S.I., Cherdantsev D.V., Vakhrunin A.A., Pervova O.V. Microcirculation of gastric and duodenal mucosa in peptic ulcer associated with Helicobacter pillory // Russian Medical Journal. -2000г. -T.4.-C. 3-5.

39. Gavrishchuk Y.V. Optimization of prophylaxis and treatment of gastrointestinal moles in victims with polytraumas. St. Petersburg, 2009

40. Gallinger YI, Gogello EA, Khrustaleva MV, Nurmanova MJ Diagnostic and therapeutic endoscopy in gastroduodenal bleeding after operations on the heart and aorta // Endoscopic Surgery. 2004. - №6. - C.39-43.

41. Hasanov Z.V., Ismayilov H.I., Rahimova L.Sh. General rules of preparation for laboratory research. Baku, 2007, 50 p.

42. Gelfand B.R., Martynov A.H., Guryanov V.A., Shipilova O.S. Prevention of stress injuries of the upper gastrointestinal tract in patients in critical conditions // Consilium medicum. Surgery. - 2004. - №2. C . 16-20.

43. Gelfand B.R., Guryanov V.A. Prevention of stress-induced damage to the gastrointestinal tract

in patients in critical conditions // Consilium medicum. 2005. - T.7, №6. - C. 464-467.

44. Govorova N.V., Voinov A.Y., Lukach V.N., et al. Damage to the vascular endothelium and disorders of the system of regulation of blood aggregate state in patients with severe craniocerebral trauma // Anesthesiology and Reanimatology, 2004,№ 6, p.32-35.

45. Goloborodko M.K. "Polgtrauma zhittovoivovazhivnyh organ is: principles of intensive therapy and intensive surgery". Odessa Medical Journal. 2004. № 4. c.4-6

46. Gostischev V.K., Evseev M.A. Acute gastroduodenal ulcer bleeding: from strategic concepts to therapeutic tactics. - M., 2005. - 352 c.

47. Gostischev V.K., Evseev M.A. New approaches to predicting recurrences of acute gastroduodenal ulcer bleeding // Vestn. Ross. akad. med. nauk. 2004. - №10. - C.26-30.

48. Guk A.P., Semisalov S.Y., Zhilyaev R.A., Kardash K.A. "Occurrence of medium-severe craniocerebral trauma during the year and day of the week in the adult population of Donetsk". Zhurn. Ukrashskiy medichniy almanac. 1'2010. C.47-48

49. Gunyat R.Ya. Acute postoperative gastroduodenal erosions and ulcers in patients with surgical lung diseases and their prevention. Dissertation. kand.med.nauk. Moscow, 2005

50. Degtyareva I.I., Skrypnik I.H., Kozachok N.N. et al. Effectiveness of the use of kvamatel in diseases of the digestive organs // Suchasna gastroenterolopia. 2002. T. 10. № 4. c. 70-77

51. Dzyak L. A., Zorin M. O., Starko A. G. "Ukrashskiy neurohsurpchnyj zhurnal" 2007,№ 3, pp. 5-6.

52. Dolina O.A. Anesthesiology and resuscitation. Textbook. Moscow. Geotar-med. 2002, 552 c.

53. Duzhiy GD. Prophylaxis of acute stress gastrostestinal virazok ta 1h ускладнень in patients with 1 spoluchenyu kran yuabdomshalnoyu trauma. GD. Duzhiy, V.P.Shevchenko, V.V.Shevchenko // Kharyuvska khrurpchna shkola. 2009.- № 4.1.-C.194-196

54. Emuzova M.S. Treatment, prognosis and prevention of acute ulceration of the stomach and duodenum in patients with chronic renal insufficiency // Author's abstract of the dissertation. Nalchik, 2003. - 21 c.

55. Ermolov A.S., Tveritneva L.F., Pakhomova G.V. et al. Gastroduodenal bleeding in critical conditions // Surgery. -2004. №8. - C.41-45.

56. Kalashnikov A.Y. Endoscopic diagnostics of mucous membrane lesions of the upper part of the gastrointestinal tract in patients with thermal burns of the body. Dissertation of Candidate of Medical Sciences - Moscow, 2005

57. Kalyagin A.N. Gastric lesions that occurred against the background of taking non-steroidal anti-inflammatory drugs // Siberian Journal of Gastroenterol. and Hepatol. 2003. - №16/17. - C. 161-162.

58. Kameneva E.A., Grigoriev E.V., Razumov A.S. et al. Optimization of diagnostics and correction of hemostasis disorders in severe craniocerebral trauma // General Resuscitation, 2007, vol. 2, No. 11, pp. 25-35.

59. Karimov R.Kh. "Epidemiologic aspects of timeliness of medical care for victims with craniocerebral trauma". Neurological Bulletin. 2006. Vol. 38, Issue 1-2, P.43-48.

60. Clinical-diagnostic significance of the most important laboratory analyses carried out in Shafa LDC. Baku, 2009, 340 p.

61. Klochkov I.N. Endoscopic characterization of lesions of the upper parts of the gastrointestinal tract in patients with hemorrhagic fever with renal syndrome, leptospirosis and tularemia. Dissertation. Cand.med.nauk - Ryazan, 2009

62. Kobiashvili M.G. Pathogenesis, prevention and correction of enteral insufficiency as a basis for a differentiated approach to nutritional support in victims with severe combined trauma. Dissertation of Candidate of Medical Sciences. St. Petersburg, 2003

63. Kobiashvili M.G., Eryukhin I.A., Shanin V.Y., Nemchenko N.S. Disorders of gastrointestinal tract organs in victims with severe trauma // Voen.-Med. zhurn. 2003. - Vol. 324, №1. - C.66-70.

64. Kozlov A.A., Kachalova N.D., Sergeeva E.V., Prostakova T.M. Manual for laboratory doctors on methods of plasma hemostasis research. Factors of blood coagulation. M., 2006, 236 pp.

65. Korshunov G. V., Korshunov A. G. Adaptation mechanisms of hemostasis / Materials of international conference on hemorheology and microcirculation. Yaroslavl, 2003, p.96.

66. Kotaev A.Y. Acute erosions and ulcers of the upper gastrointestinal tract complicated by bleeding // Russian Med. Zhurn. 2006. - T. 14, №6. - C.501-504

67. Krivosheev A. B. Gastrointestinal bleeding and their prevention in the postoperative period // Siberian Journal of Gastroenterol. and Hepatol.-2004.- № 18.-S.192-193.

68. Krylov V., Lebedev V. Craniocerebral trauma // Physician, 2000,№ 11, p.13- 21

69. Kubyshkin V.A., Shishin K.V. Erosive-ulcerous lesion of the upper parts of the gastrointestinal tract in the early postoperative period // Surgery. Consilium medicum. - 2004. - № 1. - C . 17-20.

70. Cooper L. Physics for All. Classical Physics. Volume 1 Translation from English under the editorship of Y.A.Kravtsov Moscow "Mir", 1973, 480 p., P.126-127.

71. Kurbanov H.H. Endoscopic hemostasis in gastroduodenal ulcer bleeding // Author's

dissertation. candidate of medical sciences. Dushanbe, 2002. - 20 c.

72. Latysheva V.Ya. Craniocerebral trauma, classification, clinical picture, diagnosis and treatment. Minsk: Vyshaya Shkola, 2005, 110 pp.

73. Lolenko AV, Popov AA, Sukhorukov A.M. et al. Early pathogenetic therapy of acute erosive-ulcerous lesions of the gastrointestinal tract with hemorrhage (experimental work) // Siberian Medical Journal. 2003. - T.18, №1-2. - C. 153.

74. Lutsevich E.V., Belov I.N. Treatment of ulcerative gastroduodenal bleeding: from surgery to therapy. Хирургия.-2008.-№1.-C.4-7

75. Maev IV, Samsonov AA, Busarova GA, Agapova NR Acute gastrointestinal bleeding (clinic, diagnosis, therapy) // Treating Physician. 2003. - N5. - C. 18-22.

76. Maev IV, Samsonov AA, Vyuchnova ES Gastrointestinal bleeding: modern methods of treatment // Pharmateka. 2004. - №5. - C.32-38.

77. Maev IV, Samsonov IH, Nikushkina AA Diagnosis, treatment and prevention of acute gastrointestinal bleeding //Pharmateka. 2005. - №1. - C.62-67.

78. Malyshev V.D. "Intensive care. Resuscitation. First aid. Moscow "Medicine". 2000, 420 c.

79. Malyshev V.D. "Intensive therapy" manual for doctors. Moscow "Medicine". 2002. 584 c.

80. Mandel A.A. Acute erosive-ulcerous lesions of the stomach and duodenum at the pathology of biliary tract // Author's disc. candidate of medical sciences. M., 2004. -23 c.

81. Matlina E.S. To the question about the participation of catecholamines in the organism of stress reactions. Physiology and biochemistry of mediator processes. Moscow: 1996, pp. 74-75

82. Matlina E.Sh. About determination of adrenaline and noradrenaline in blood / Works on new equipment and methods of the 1st Moscow Medical Institute, M., 1985, Vyp. 3, c. 84-87

83. Matchin EN, Marysheva TE, Khadartsev AA Erosive-ulcerous lesions of the gastrointestinal tract in burned // Vestn. new medical technol. 2003. - №1/2. - C.68-70.

84. Mashkovsky M.D. Medicines: Guide for doctors. 15th ed. Moscow. Novaya volna. 2005, c.633-634.

85. T.A. Morozova Hypothalamic syndrome. Military Academy. Volgograd city.

86. Neurosurgery (normative documents of the Ministry of Health of Ukraine). 2004-2008.- K: Vshol, 2009, 265 p.

87. Nikiforov PA, Belousova EA Place quamatel (famotidine) in the therapy of erosive-ulcerous

lesions of the upper gastrointestinal tract //Medicine. 2004. - №2. - C.94-95.

88. Nikiforov PA, Bazarova MA, Nikitina SA Application of H2-blockers in bleeding from gastroduodenal ulcers and prevention of their development // Med. panorama. 2005. - №5. - C.40-41.

89. Osadchiy V.A. Morphologic and pathogenetic features of gastroduodenal ulcers in elderly patients with myocardial infarction // Clinich. gerontology. 2004. - T. 10, №7. - C. 9-14.

90. Osipov I.S. Damage to the mucous membrane of the gastrointestinal tract in the wounded and injured with multiple and combined trauma. Dissertation of Candidate of Medical Sciences, 121 p.

91. Pedachenko E.G., Shlapak I.P., Ruk A.P., Pilipenko M.N. "Craniocerebral trauma: modern principles of emergency care: Educational method. manual. Kiev. Vipol. 2009. 216 c.

92. Polushin Y.S. et al. "Manual of Anesthesiology and Reanimatology". St. Petersburg. "ELBI-SPb" 2004, 720 pp.

93. Poputchikova E.A. Acute erosions and ulcers of the stomach and duodenum complicated by bleeding in patients with myocardial infarction. Avtoref. dis. kand. med. nauk. M., 2003. - 26 c.

94. Ryabkova AA, Shostak NA, Malyarova LP Gastrointestinal bleeding due to taking non-steroidal anti-inflammatory drugs // Physician. 2004. - №4. - C.26-27.

95. Samoday V.G., Shagivaleev N.A. Posttraumatic "stress ulcers" of the stomach and duodenum as a complication of severe combined, multiple and combined traumas. /Department of Traumatology, Orthopedics and Military Field Surgery of the State Educational Institution of Higher Professional Education VPO VGMA named after N.N. Burdenko of Roszdrav.

96. Sadritdinov M.A. Diagnostics and treatment of intestinal insufficiency syndrome in patients with widespread peritonitis. Dissertation of Candidate of Medical Sciences Ufa, 2006

97. Smirnova L.E. Features of microcirculation in the gastric mucosa at gastroduodenal pathology. Morphology. 2004. T.126. Vyp. 4, C. 114

98. Sokolov V.A. Multiple and combined traumas. Publisher: GEOTAR-media. 2006, S.Mon., 518 p.

99. Spiridonova T.G. Poliorgan dysfunction and insufficiency in burned people. Dissertation of Candidate of Medical Sciences. Moscow, 2007

100. Stoyko Y. M., Kurygin A. A. A. A., Musinov I. M. Vagotomy in the treatment of acute gastric ulceration complicated by severe bleeding // Vestn. of Surgery. 2001. - №3. - C.25-29.

101. Strekalovsky VP, Shishin KV, Starkov YG, Domarev JI.B.. Bleeding from the upper parts of the gastrointestinal tract after operations on the abdominal cavity // Surgery. 2004. - №8. -C.7680.

102. Stukalenko D.O. Prediction, prevention and treatment of acute erosions and ulcers of the mucous membrane of the gastrointestinal tract in wounded and injured. Dissertation. Cand. Med. Nauk. St. Petersburg. 2008, 116 c.

103. Stukalenko D.O. Prediction of formation, complications and localization of acute erosions and ulcers of the mucous membrane in wounded and injured patients.- St. Petersburg, 2007. - T. 10, №7. - C. 9-14.

104. Stukalenko D.O. Pathology: prevention and treatment of acute erosions and ulcers of the gastrointestinal tract in the wounded and injured: autoref. dis. . cand. med. sciences. St. Petersburg, 2008, 14 p.

105. Timerbulatov V.M., Hasanov A.G., Sadritdinov M.A. Significance of ischemia-reperfusion in the occurrence of erosive and ulcerative lesions of the gastroduodenal zone // Annals of Surgery. 2003. - №3. - C. 49-53.

106. Tikhonov V.I., Popov O.S., Shpilevoy P.K. et al. Acute ulcer bleeding in the clinic of general surgery // Siberian Journal of Gastroenterol. and Hepatol. 2004. - №18. - C. 77-79.

107. Unzhakov V.V., Kondratyev A.N. Sedation and study of the dynamics of some hormones in the early postoperative period in patients with severe craniocerebral trauma // Anesthesiology and Reanimatology, 2005,№ 4, p.52-55.

108. Urazbakhtin I.M.Endoscopic methods and mini-invasive technologies in diagnostics and complex treatment of urgent diseases and traumas of abdominal cavity organs (experimental and clinical study). Dissert. kand. med. nauk. Ufa, 2005

109. Fazulin B.P., Amcheslavsky V.G., Iskhanov O.S. et al. Principles of intensive therapy in the acute period of severe craniocerebral trauma in children /Anesthesiology and Reanimatology, 2000,№ 4, p. 57 - 59

110. "Human Physiology" 4 vols. 4th volume, section 26, 29. Translation from English by N.N.Alipov, V.L.Bykov and B.A.Konnikov, edited by Acad. P.K.Kostyuk, pp.109-143, 221-265.

111. Khaliullin AI, Pikovsky V.I., Dodelia V.Sh. Medikamentoznaya prophylaxis of stress ulcers of the gastrointestinal tract //Medicine critical states. 2005. - №8. - C.52-57.

112. Kharkin A.V., Lobacheva G.V., Manerova A.F. et al. Prevention and treatment of gastroduodenal bleeding in pediatric cardiac surgery // Anesthesiology and resuscitation. 2005. - №1. - C. 38-41.

113. Tsarenko S.V. Neuroreanimatology. Intensive therapy of craniocerebral trauma. Moscow: Medicine, 2006, p.231 -233.

114. Tsarenko S.V. Modern approaches to intensive therapy of severe craniocerebral trauma //Anesthesiology and Reanimatology, 2003,№ 2, p.45-49.

115. Tsurupa S.D. Comparative evaluation of endoscopic methods of hemostasis in bleeding from the upper parts of the gastrointestinal tract // Author's Dissertation of Candidate of Medical Sciences. St. Petersburg, 2004. - 18 c.

116. Chernobrovy V.M., Chernova I.V., Meleshchenko S.G.. "Dan! ekspregastro pH-metrn yak kriteritsh starterovoyu recognizatsii blocka - tor!v N+K+ATP-azi pri virazkovsh khvorov! schloroduodenalnogo localhzatsn" Suchasna gastrostroterologiologiia! 2004,№ 1, p.29-33

117. Chernov A.L., Feskov A.E. "Methodological bases of diagnostic protocols and treatment of combined craniocerebral trauma at the prehospital stage". Zhurnal Khark'vsko kh!rurg'chna shkola. 1'2010, c.46-48

118. Chernousov A.F., Khorobrykh T.V., Urzhumtseva G.A., Urakova Ya. Endoscopic hemostasis of erosive-ulcer gastroduodenal bleeding with the use of fibrin glue in patients in critical condition // Surgery. 2006. - №8. - c. 17-20.

119. Shagivaleev N.A., Samoday V.G. Acute ("stress") ulcers of the gastrointestinal tract in patients with craniocerebral trauma. / Department of Traumatology, Orthopedics and Military Field Surgery of GOU VPO VGMA named after N.N. Burdenko Roszdrav.

120. Shapkin Yu.G., Maslyakova G.N., Kapralov S.V. et al. Laser photocoagulation of bleeding gastric and duodenal ulcer // Surgery. 2006. -№5. C.23-25.

121. Shilova E.A. Acute gastroduodenal bleeding as a complication of the immediate postoperative period in patients who have undergone surgical interventions on the heart and blood vessels // Author's dissertation of Candidate of Medical Sciences. M., 2003. - 27 c.

122. Shlevkov VA, Abramova LA, Toguzova DA Experience of clinical use of quamatel in bleeding from the upper parts of the gastrointestinal tract // Surgery. 2001. - №7. - C.45-48.

123. Shostak NA, Ryabkova AA, Savelyev VS, Malyarova LP Gastrointestinal bleeding as complications of gastropathy associated with the use of nonsteroidal anti-inflammatory drugs // Terapevtich. archive. 2003. - №5. - C.70-73.

124. Aitkenhead AP, Smith G. Guide to anesthesiology and resuscitation. Moscow. "Medicine". Vol. 1 -2. 2010, 810 c.

125. Yashchenko V.I. Endoscopic vagotomy in complex treatment and prevention of stress gastroduodenal ulcers. Dissertation. kand.med.nauk. Moscow, 2004

126. Abe Y., Jnamori M., Togova J.I. et al. The comparative effects of single intravenous doses of

omeprazole end famotidine on intragastric pH // J. Gastroenterol. Gastroenterol. 2004. - Vol.39, №1. - P.21-25.

127. Adamopoulos AB, Baibas NM, Efstathiou SP, Tsioulos DI, Mitromaras AG, Tsami AA, Mountokalakis TD. Differentiation between patients wih acute upper gastrointestinal bleeding who need early urgent upper gastrointestinal endoscopy and those who do not. A prospective study. Eur J Gastroenterol Hepatol 2003; 15:381-387.

128. Al-Balbissi AH. Role of gender in road accidents. Traffic Inj Prev 2003;4:64-73.

129. Akhtar AJ, Ganesan K, Yoshikawa TT. Upper gastrointestinal hemorrhage in African-American and Hispanic elderly patients. Ethn Dis 2001;11:7-10.

130. Akinci H, Yucel T, Kuroglu E, Gurdal SO. Evaluation criteria for selecting patients for surgical or nonoperative treatment in nonvariceal upper gastrointestinal bleeding. Ulus Travma Dergisi 2004;10:226-231.

131. Aljebreen AM, Fallone CA, Barkun A. Nasogastric aspirate predicts high-risk endoscopic lesions in patients with acute upper-GI bleeding. Gastrointest Endosc 2004; 59(2):172-178.

132. Arabi Y, Al Knawy B, Barkun AN, et al. Procon debate: octreotide has an important role in the treatment of gastrointestinal bleeding of unknown origin? Crit Care. 2006; 10(4):218.

133. Archimandritis A, Tsirantonaki M, Tryphonos M, et al. Ranitidine versus ranitidine plus octreotide in the treatment of acute non-variceal upper gastrointestinal bleeding: a prospective randomized study. Curr Med Res Opm. 2000;16(3):178-83.

134. Arlt G.D,Leyh M: Incidence an pathophysiology of peptic ulcer bleeding.Langenbeck's Arch Surg 2001;386:75-81

135. Banoob D.W., McCloskey W.W. Webster W. Risk of gastric injury with enteric- versus nonenteric-coated aspirin // Ann. Pharmacother. 2002. - Vol.36, №1.-P.163-166.

136. Bardou M, Youssef M, Toubouti Y, et al. Newer endoscopic therapies decrease both re-bleeding and mortality in high risk patients with acute peptic ulcer bleeding: a series of meta-analyses.Gastroenterology. 2003; 123:239.

137. Bardou M, Toubouti Y, Benhaberou-Brun D, et al. High dose proton pump inhibition decreases both re-bleeding and mortality in high-risk patients with acute peptic ulcer bleeding. A series of metaanalyses. Gastroenterology. 2003; 123:625.

138. Barkun A, Bardou M, Marshall JK. Consensus recommendations for managing patients with nonvariceal upper gastrointestinal bleeding. Ann Intern Med 2003; 139(10):843-857.

139. Barkun A, Fallone CA, Chiba N. A Canadian clinical practice algorithm for the management of patients with nonvariceal upper gastrointestinal bleeding. Can J Gastroenterol 2004; 18(10):605-609.

140. Barkun A, Sabbah S, Enns R, Armstrong D, Gregor J, Fedorak RNN, Rahme E, Toubouti Y, Martel M, Chiba N, Fallone CA. The Canadian Registry on Nonvariceal Upper Gastrointestinal Bleeding and Endoscopy (RUGBE): Endoscopic hemostasis and proton pump inhibition are associatede with improved outcomes in a real life setting. Am J Gastroenterol. 2004; 99 (7): 1238.

141. Bass BL, Turner DJ. Acute gastrointestinal hemorrhage. Towsend CM (ed). Sabiston Textbook of Surgery. 17th edition. Philedelphia: Saunders Company; 2004. 1244-1255.

142. Bayir A, Okumuş M. Üst gis kanamalarmda risk faktorlerininin prognoz üzerine etkisi. Genel Tip Derg 2003;13:157-61.

143. Belaiche J, Burette A, De Vos M, Louis E, Huybrechts M, Deltenre M; Belgian Study Group of NSAID- GI Complications. Observational survey of NSAID-related upper gastrointestinal adverse events in Belgium. Acta Gastroenterol Belg. 2002 Apr-Jun; 65(2): 65-73.

144. Bener A, Ozkan T, Lajunen T. The Driver Behavior Questionnaire in Arab Gulf countries: Qatar and United Arab Emirates. Accid Anal Prev 2008;40:1411-7.

145. Bener A. The neglected epidemic: road traffic accidents in a developing country, State of Qatar. Int J Inj ontr Saf Promot 2005;12:45-7.

146. Bener A, Crundall D. Road traffic accidents in the United Arab Emirates compared to western countries. Adv Transport Stud Int J 2005;6:5- 12.

147. Bener A, Ghaffar A, Azab A, Sankaran-Kutty M, Toth F, Lovasz G. The impact of four-wheel drives on traffic disability and deaths compared to passenger cars. J Coll Physicians Surg Pak 2006;16:257-60.

148. Bener A, Lajunen T, Ozkan T, Haigney D, The effect of mobile phone use on driving style and driving skills. Int J Crashworthiness 2006;11:459-65.

149. Bener A. Emerging Trend in Motorization and the Epidemic of Road Traffic Crashes in an Economically Growing Country. International Journal of Crashworthiness 2009 (In the press).

150. Bener A, Crundall D. Effects of driver behavior on accident involvement: The role of gender and driver behavior in Road Traffic Crashes. Int J Crashworthiness 2008;13:331-6.

151. Bener A, Al-Maadid M, Ozkan T, Al-Bast DAE, Diyab KN, Lajunen T. The impact of four wheel driver on risky driver behaviors and road traffic accidents. Transportation Research Intl Journal Part F: Traffic Psychy & Behaviour 2008A;324-33.

152. Bjorkman DJ, Zaman A, Fennerty MB, Lieberman D, DiSario JA, GuestWarnick G. Urgent vs. elective endoscopy for acute non-variceal upper GI bleeding: an effectiveness study. Gastrointest Endosc 2004; 60(1):1-8

153. Blalia V., Simek J., Zadak Z., Sobotka L. Medium chain triglycerides versus long chain triglycerides in nutritional support of liver regeneration // J. Clin. Clin. Nutr. and Gastroenterology - 2001. -Vol. 6. №1.-P.l 1-17.

154. Blatchford O, Murray WR, Blatchford M. A risk score to predict need for treatment for upper gastrointestinal hemorrhage. Lancet 2000; 356:13181321.

155. Blocksom JM, Tokioka S, Sugawa C.Current therapy for nonvariceal upper gastrointestinal bleeding. Surg Endosc.2004;18(2):186-92.

156. Boonpongmanee S, Fleischer DE, Pezzullo JC, Collier K, Mayoral W, Al- Kawas F, Chutkan R, Lewis JH, Tio TL, Benjamin SB. The frequency of peptic ulcer as a cause of upper-GI bleeding is exaggerated. Gastrointest Endosc 2004;59:788-794.

157. Borrell *C,* Plasència A, Huisman M, Costa G, Kunst A, Andersen O, et al. Education level inequalities and transportation injury mortality in the middle aged and elderly in European settings. Inj Prev 2005;11:138-42.

158. Bolondi L., Gaiani S. Gall bladder sluge formation during prolonged fasting after gastrointestinal track surgery // Gut. -2005.-Vol.26. no.7.-P.734-738.

159. Bowling T.E., Silk D.B.A. Pathophysiology of diarrhoea and the role of fiber in enteral nutrition // Clin. Nutr. -2005. -Vol.14, Suppl.l.-P.84-86.

160. Burnham W.R. Nutritional support of patients witla gastrointestinal disease // Brit. J. Clin. Pharmacol. -2002. -Vol.14. №3. -P.315-324.

161. Bozzetti F. Home total parenteral nutrition in cancer patients // Clin. Nutr. - 2005.Vol.14, Suppl.l. -P.36-40.

162. Bozzetti F. Perioperative nutrition: the rationale for nutritional support //Clin. Nutr. -2003. -Vol.15. No. 4.-P. 155-156.

163. Brinson R., Guild R., Kolts B. Diarrhea and hypoalbimiinemia in a medical intensive care unit// Gastroenterology. -2005. -Vol. 88. №5. -P.1336.

164. British Society of Gastroenterology Endoscopy Committee. Non-variceal upper gastrointestinal haemorrhage: guidelines. Gut. 2002; 51(4):iv1-6.

165. Brullet E, Campo R, Calvet X, Guell M, Garcia-Monforte N, Cabrol J. A randomized study of

the safety of outpatient care for patients with bleeding peptic ulcer treated by endoscopic injection. Gastrointest Endosc 2004; 60(1):15-21.

166. Bustamante M, Stollman N. The efficacy of proton-pump inhibitors in acute ulcer bleeding: a qualitative review // J. Clin. Clin. Gastroenterol. 2000. Vol.30, №1.-P.7-13.

167. Buzby G.P., Mullen J.L., Mattews D.C. et al. Prognostic nutritional index in gastrointestinal surgery // Am. J. Surg. -2000. -Vol.139. no. 1. -P. 160-166.

168. Caban A., Wiaderkiewicz R., Kaminski M., et al. Arterial ketone index in assessing liver function and its detoxicative capability after ischemiareperfusion injury // Acta Biochim Pol. 2000. V. 47. № 4. P. 1137-1146.

169. Castell D.O., Kahrilas P.J., Richter J.E.. Esomeprazole (40 mg) compared with lansoprazole (30 mg) in the tretment of erosive oesophagitis //Amer J Gastroenterol. 2002. V. 97. P. 575-583.

170. Camellini L. Comparison of three different risk scoring systems in non- variceal upper gastrointestinal bleeding. Dig Liver Dis 2004; 36(4):271-277 (Abstract).

171. Cameron E.A., Pratap J.N., Sims T.J., et al. Three-year prospective validation of a pre-endoscopic risk stratification in patients with acute upper gastrointestinal haemorrhage /Eur J Gastroenterol Hepatol. 2002. May. V. 14. №5. P. 497-501.

172. Candelli M, Nista EC, Carloni E, et al. Treatment of H. Pylori infection : A review Current Medicinal Chemistry 2005;12:375-84.

173. Candusso M, Giglio L., Faraguna D. Long-term home parenteral nutrition in children// Clin. Nutr. -2001. -Vol.14. Suppl.l. -P.28-32.

174. Carlson G., Maqeure G. Quality of life on home parenteral nutrition: a single center study of 37 patients // Clin. Nutr.-2005.-Vol. 14. №4.-P.219-228.

175. Catala I, Juste C, Benfiguig K. et al. Use of soy proteins in cholelithiasis prevention // Second international symposium on the role of soy in preventing and treating chronic disease. Brussels, 2003. -P. 16.

176. Cederholm T.E., Hellstrom K.H.. Reversibility of protein-energy malnutrition in a group of chronically-ill elderly outpatients // Clin. Nutr.- 2005.-Vol.14. No.2. -P.81-87.

177. Chan FKL, Wu CY, et al. Eradication of HP and the risk of peptic ulcers in patients starting on long - term treatment with NSAIDs: a randomized trial. Lancet 2002;359:9-13.

178. Chandra R.K.. 2000 McCollum award lecture. Nutrition and immunity lessons from the past and new insights into the future // Am. J. Clin. Nutr.- 2001. -Vol.53, No.5.-P.1087-1101.

179. Chey WD, Scheiman JM. Peptic Ulcer Disease. In: Friedman SL, McQuaid KR, Grendell JH, eds. Diagnosis and Treatment in Gastroenterology. 2nd ed: McGraw-Hill 2003. p.323-42

180. Church NI, Palmer KR. Relevance of the Rockall score in patients undergoing endoscopic therapy for peptic ulcer haemorrhage. Eur J Gastroenterol Hepatol 2001; 13:1149-1152.

181. Cipolletta L, Bianco MA, Rotondano G, Marmo R, Piscopo R. Outpatient management for low-risk nonvariceal upper GI bleeding: A randomized controlled trial. Gastrointest Endosc 2002; 55(1): 1 -5.

182. Conrad S.A. Acute upper gastrointestinal bleeding in critically ill patients: causes and treatment modalities // Crit Care Med. 2002. Jun. V. 30. № 6. P. 365-373.

183. Cook D.J., Griffit L.E., Walter S.D. et al. The attributable mortality and length of intensive care unit stay of clinically impotent gastrointestinal bleeding in critically ill pacients // Crit. Care. 2001. -№5. - P.368-375.

184. Cosnes J. Oral and enteral nutrition management and drug treatment of short bowel syndrome // Clin. Nutr. -2005. -Vol.14. Suppl.l -P. 16-20.

185. Courtney AE, Mitchell RMS, Rocke L, Johnston BT. Proposed risk stratification in upper gastrointestinal haemorrhage: Is hospitalization essential. Emerg Med J 2004; 21:39-40.

186. Daley R.J., Rebuck J.A., Welag L.S., Rogers F.B.. Prevention of stress ulceration: current trends in critical care // Crit Care Med. 2004. V. 32. № 10. P. 2008-2021.

187. Das A, Wong RCK. Prediction of outcome of acute GI hemorrhage: a review of risk scores and predictive models. Gastrointest Endosc 2004; 60(1):85-93.

188. De Caestecker J.Upper Gastrointestinal Bleeding: Surgical Perspective. Medicine 2002; 9:1 33.

189. De Francesco A., Maffi G. et al. Home parenteral nutrition in Italy: data from the Italian National Register //Clin. Nutr. -2005. -Vol.14. Supl.l. -P.69.

190. Defreyne L, Vanlangenhove P, De Vos M, et al. Embolization as a first approach with endoscopically unmanageable acute nonvariceal gastrointestinal hemorrhage. Radiology. 2001; 218(3):739-48.

191. De Ledinghen V., Beau P., Labat J., Ingrand P. Compared effects of enteral nutrition by percutaneous endoscopic gastrostomy in cancer and in noncancer patients: a long-term study // Clin. Nutr. -2005. -Vol.14. №1. -P. 1722.

192. Depolo A, Dobrila-Dintinjana R, Uravi M, et all. Upper gastrointestinal bleeding - Review of our ten years results. Zentralbl Chir 2001; 126: 772776.

193. De Wit L.M., Nieboer M., Wipkink A. et al. Differences betwe hospitals in home enteral nutrition//Clin. Nutr. -2005. -Vol.14. Suppl.2.-P.42.

194. Di Fiore F, Lecleire S, Merl V, et al. Changes in characteristics and outcome of acute upper gastrointestinal haemorrhage: a comparison of epidemiology and practices between 1996 and 2000 in a multicentre French study. European Journal of Gastroenterology & Hepatology 2005; 6: 641-7.

195. Dimmitt L, Dimmitt S, Wilson G. Diagnosis of gastrointestinal bleeding in adults. Am Fam Physician 2005; 71: 1339-1346.

196. Dionigi R., Dominioni L. Perioperative nutritional support in cancer pa- tient//Bibliot. Nutr. et Dieta. -2003. -№35. -P.85-94.

197. Ditschuneit H., Faulhaber J.D., Beil I., Pfeiffer E.F.. Veranderung des Stoffwechsels bei Null-Diat // Internist. -2000. -Jg. 11. H.5. -S.176-183.

198. Douglass A, Bramble MG, Barrison I. National survey of UK emergency endoscopy units. BMJ 2005;330(7498):1000-1001

199. Dudrick S.J.. Past, present and future of nutritional support // Surg. Clin. North. Am. -2001. -Vol.71. №3. -P.439-448.

200. Duggan AE, Logan RPH. Helicobacter pylori: Diagnosis and Management. In: Bloom S, ed. Practical Gastroenterology. London: Martin Dunitz Ltd 2002. p.471-84.

201. Dunlin G.A., Fidanza F. Evaluation of nutritional status // Bibliot. Nutr. et Dieta. -2005. -№ 35. -P.20-30.

202. Dulai GS, Gralnek IM, Oei TT, Chang D, Alofaituli G, Gornbein J, Kahn K. Utilization of health care resources for low-risk patients with acute, nonvariceal upper GI hemorrhage: An historical cohort study. Gastrointest Endosc 2002; 55(3):321-327.

203. Dursun M, Yilmaz S, Yikselen V, Canoru3 F, Tuzcu A. Analysis of 1242 cases with upper gastrointestinal system bleeding in Southeastern Turkey: a different etiologic spectrum. Hepatogastroenterology. 2005;52:1456-1458.

204. Dworzak F., Gavazzi C et al. Effect of cancer cachexia on muscle and total body protein turnover // Clin. Nutr.-2003.-Vol. 14. Suppl.2. -P.4243.

205. Dworzak F., Ferrari P., Gavazzi C et al. Effect of total parenteral nutrition on muscle and whole body protein turnover in cancer cachexia // Clin. Nutr.2004. -Vol.14, Suppl.2. -P.38-39.

206. Erstad B.L.. Cost-effectiveness of proton pump inhibitor therapy for acute peptic ulcer-related bleeding //Crit Care Med. 2004. V. 32. № 6. P. 12771283.

207. Fan S.T., Lo CM., Lai E.C.S. et al. Perioperative nutritional support in patients undergoing hepatectomy for hepatocellular carcinoma // New Eng. J. Med. 2004. -Vol.331. №23.-P.1547-1552.

208. Felig D.M., Carafa C.J.. Stress ulcers of the stomach // Gastrointest. Endosc. 2000. - Vol.51, No.5. - P.596.

209. Fennerty M.B.. Pathophysiology of the upper gastrointestinal tract in the critically ill patient: Rationale for the therapeutic benefits of acid suppression //Crit Care Med. 2002. V. 30(6). P. 351-355.

210. Fiaccadori E., Maggiore U., Clima B., Melfa L., Rottelli c., Borghetti A. Incidence, risk factors, and prognosis of gastrointestinal hemorrhage complicating acute renal failure // Kidney Internat. 2001. - Vol. 59, №4. -P.1 510-1519.

211. Franciosi C.M., Romano F., Caprotti R.; Uggeri F. Multiple gastric perforations in an immunodepressed child. // Surgery. 2002. - Vol.131, No.6. -P.685-686.

212. Gallitelli L. Trace element and vitamin requirements in patients receiving parenteral nutrition// Clin. Nutr. -2003. -Vol. 14. Suppl.l. -P.70-74.

213. Garripoli A, Mondardini A, Turco D, Martinoglio P, Secreto P, Ferrari A. Hospitalization for peptic ulcer bleeding: evaluation of a risk scoring system in clinical practice. Dig Liver Dis 2000; 32(7):577-582 (Abstract).

214. Gisbert JP, Gonzalez L, Calvet X, Roque M, Gabriel R, Pajares JM. Proton pump inhibitors versus H2-antagonists : a meta-analysis of their efficacy in treating bleeding peptic ulcer. Aliment Pharmacol Ther. 2001;15:917-26.

215. Gisbert JP, Liorca I, Cantero J, Pajares JM. Clinical and endoscopic prognostic factors in patients with bleeding ulcer. Med Clin (Barc). 2002 Apr 13;118(13):481-6.

216. Gralnek IM, Dulai GS. Incremental value of upper endoscopy for triage of patients with acute non-variceal upper-GI hemorrhage. Gastrointest Endosc 2004; 60(1):9-14 (Abstract).

217. Gralnek IM. Outpatient management of low-risk nonvariceal upper GI hemorrhage. Are we ready to put evidence into practice. Gastrointest Endosc 2002; 55(1):131-134.

218. Gunay K, Cabioglu N, Barbaros U, et al. Endoscopic ligation for patients with active bleeding Mallory-Weiss tears. Surg Endosc. 2001; 15(11):1305- 7. Epub 2001 Sep 4.

219. Hamoui N, Docherty SD, Crookes PF. Gastrointestinal hemorrhage: is the surgeon obsolete. Emerg Med Clin North Am 2003; 21(4):1017-1056.

220. Hernandez-Diaz S,Garcia-Rodriguez L.A: Incidence of serious upper gastrointestinal

bleeding/perforation in the general population:Review of epidemiologic studies.J Clin Epidemiol 2002;55:157-163

221. Hiramoto J.S. Evidence-based analysis: postoperative gastric bleeding: etiology and prevention // Surgical Oncology. 2003. V. 12. P. 9-19.

222. Hochain P, Capet C, Colin R. Digestive complications of aspirin. Rev Med Interne 2000;21:50-9.

223. Huang CS, Lichtenstein DR. Nonvariceal upper gastrointestinal bleeding.Gastroenterol Clin North Am. 2003; 32(4):1053-1078.

224. Jensen DM, Kovacs TO, Jutabha R, et al. Randomized trial of medical or endoscopic therapy to prevent recurrent ulcer hemorrhage in patients with adherent clots. Gastroenterology. 2002; 123: 407-13.

225. Jani PG. Dieulafoy's lesion; a case report. East Afr Med J. 2001;78:109-110.

226. Jung HK, Son HY, Jung SA, et al. Comparison of oral omeprazole and endoscopic ethanol injection therapy for prevention of recurrent bleeding from peptic ulcers with nonbleeding visible vessels or fresh adherent clots. Am J Gastroenterol. 2002; 97: 1736-40.

227. Jutabha R, Jensen DM. Acute upper gastrointestinal bleeding. In: Friedman SL, McQuaid KR, Grendell JH (eds). Current Diagnosis & Treatment in Gastroenterology. 2nd ed. New York: McGraw-Hill Co, 2003: 53-69.

228. Kaplan RC, Heckbert SR, Psaty BM. Risk factors for hospitalized upper or lower gastrointestinal tract bleeding intreated hypertensives. Prev Med 2002;34:455-62.

229. Kasadipidis P, Georgopoulos P, Delis V, et al. Endoscopic management and long term follow up of Dieulafoy's lesions in the upper GI tract.Gastrointestinal Endoscopy. 2002;55:527-31.

230. Khuroo MS, Khuroo MS, Farahat KL, Kagevi IE. Treatment with proton pump inhibitors in acute non-variceal upper gastrointestinal bleeding: A meta-analysis. J Gastroenterol Hepatol 2005; 20:11-25.

231. Klebl F, Bregenzer N, Schpfer L, Tamme W, Langgartner J, Schplmerich J, Messmann H. Risk factors for mortality in severe upper gastrointestinal bleeding. Int J Colorectal Dis 2005; 20:49-56.

232. Kullavanuaya P, Manotaya S, Thong-Ngam D, et al. Efficacy of octreotide in the control of acute upper gastrointestinal bleeding. J Med Assoc Thai. 2001;84(12):1714-20

233. Kortas DY, Haas LS, Simpson WG, et al. Mallory-Weiss tear: predisposing factors and predictors of a complicated course.Am J Gastroenterol. 2001; 96(10):2863-5

234. Kwan V, Bourke MJ, Williams SJ et al. Argon plasma coagulation in the management of symptomatic gastrointestinal vascular lesions: experience in 100 consecutive patients with long-term follow-up. Am. J. Gastroenterol. 2006; 101: 58-63.

235. Kwan V, Norton ID. Endoscopic management of non-variceal upper gastrointestinal haemorrhage. ANZ J Surg. 2007;77(4):222-30.

236. Lai KC, Hui WM, Wong WM, et al. Treatment of Helicobacter pylori in patients with duodenal ulcer hemorrhage-a long-term randomized, controlled study. Am J Gastroenterol. 2000; 95:2225-32.

237. Lamberts R., Brunner G., Solcia E. Effects of very long (up to 10 years) proton pump blockade on human gastric mucosa // Digestion. 2001. V. 64. №4. P. 205-213.

238. Lanas A, Bajador E, Serrano P, et al. Nitrovasodilators, low-dose aspirin, other nonsteroidal anti-inflammatory drugs, and the risk of upper gastrointestinal bleeding. N Engl J Med 2000; 384: 834.

239. Lau JY, Sung JJ, Lee KK, et al. Effect of intravenous omeprazole on recurrent bleeding after endoscopic treatment of bleeding peptic ulcers. N Engl J Med. 2000; 343: 310-316

240. Lau JYW, Chung SCS. Hematemesis and melena. Weinstein W, Hawkey C, Bosch J (ed). Clinical gastroenterology and hepatology. 1.st ed. Philadelphia: Mosby; 2004. 112-118.

241. Lee JG. Urgent endoscopy: does it matter if they don't listen to us. Gastrointest Endosc 2004; 60(1):94-95.

242. Lefkovitz Z, Cappell MS, Kaplan M, Mitty H, Gerard P. Radiology in the diagnosis and therapy of gastrointestinal bleeding. Gastroenterol Clin North Am 2000; 29:489-512

243. Leontiadis GI, Sreedharan A, Dorward S, et al. Systematic reviews of the clinical effectiveness and cost-effectiveness of proton pump inhibitors in acute upper gastrointestinal bleeding. Health Technol Assess. 2007; 11(51):1-164

244. Leontiadis G.I., Sharma V.K., Howden C.W.. Proton pump ingibitor treatment for acute peptic ulcer bleeding // Cochrane Database syst. Rev. - 2006. Vol.25, No.1. - CD 002094.

245. Lewis J.D., Shin E.J., Metz D.C. Characterization of gastrointestinal bleeding in severely ill hospitalized patients // Crit. Care Med. 2000. - Vol.28, №1. - P.46-50.

246. Lewis J.D., Kimmel S.E., Localio A.R., Metz D.C. et al. Risk of serious upper gastrointestinal toxicity with over-the-counter nonaspirin nosteroidal anti-inflammatory drugs // Gastroenterology. 2005. - Vol.129, No.6. -P. 18651874.

247. Linhares MM, Filho BH, Schraibman V, et al. Dieulafoy lesion: endoscopic and surgical

management. Surg Laparosc Endosc Endosc Percutan Tech. 2006; 16(1):1-3

248. Llach J, Elizalde JI, Guevara MC, et al. Endoscopic injection therapy in bleeding Mallory-Weiss syndrome: a randomized controlled trial. Gastrointest Endosc.2001; 54(6):679-81

249. Lye CC, Jeremy GC. Scoring systems and risk assessment for upper gastrointestinal bleeding. Eur J Gastroenterol Hepatol 2001; 13(10):1137- 1139.

250. Maltfertheiner P, Megraud F, O'Morain F, et al. European Helicobacter Pylori Study Group. Current concepts in management of Helicobacter pylori infection-the Maastricht 2-2000 Concensus Report. Aliment Pharmacol Ther 2002;16:167-80.

251. Maltz C. Acute gastrointestinal bleeding. Best Practice of Medicine. February 2003: 1-19.

252. Marik P.E., Zaloga G.P. Early enteral nutrition in acutely ill patients: a systematic review // Crit Care Med. 2001. - Vol.29, No.6 - P.2264-2270.

253. Marmo R, Rotondano G, Bianco MA, et al. Outcome of endoscopic treatment for peptic ulcer bleeding: Is a second look necessary? A metaanalysis. Gastrointest Endosc. 2003; 57(1):62-7.

254. McLaren R., Jarvis C.L., Fish D.N.. Use of enteral nutrition for stress ulcer prophylaxis // Ann Pharmacother. 2001. - Vol.35, No.4 - P.1614-1623.

255. Mellemkjaer L, Blot WJ, Sorensen HT, Thomassen L, McLaughlin JK, Nielsen GL, Olsen JH. Upper gastrointestinal bleeding among users of NSAIDs: a population-based cohort study in Denmark. Br J Clin Pharmacol. 2002 Feb; 53(2):173-81.

256. Mellinger JD. Upper gastrointestinal endoscopy: current status. Semin Laparosc Surg 2003;10:3-12.

257. Miller FH, Hwang CM. An initial experience: using helical CT imaging to detect obscure gastrointestinal bleeding. Clin Imaging 2004; 28:245-251.

258. Mostafa G., Sing R.F., Matthews B.D., Pratt B.L., Norton H.J., Heni- ford.B.T.. The economic benefit of practice guidelines for stress ulcer prophylaxis // Am. Surg. 2002. - Vol.68, №1. - P. 146-150.

259. Monturo Ch.A. Enteral access device selection // Nutr. Clin. Pract. -2000.- Vol.5, No.5.-P.207-213.

260. Morimoto T., Tsujinaka T., Kishibuchi M. et al. Down regulation of albumin synthesis by continouos parenteral nutrition and its modulation by cyclic parenteral nutrition // Clin. Nutr. -2005. -Vol.14. Suppl.2.-P.20.

261. Mumtaz R. Outcomes of endoscopic treatment of gastroduodenal Dieulafoy's lesion with rubber

band ligation and thermal/injection therapy. J Clin Gastroenterol 2003; 36(4):310-314 (Abstract).

262. Mutlu G.M., Mutlu E.A. Factor P-Gl complicatious in patients receiving mechanical ventilation // Chest. 2001. - Vol. 119. - P. 1222-1241.

263. Oh DS, Pisegna JR. Management of upper gastrointestinal bleeding. Clin Fam Pract 2004; 6(3):631-645.

264. Oh YJ. Clinical usefulness of Rockall scoring system in patients with bleeding peptic ulcer--comparison with Forrest classification. Korean J Gastroenterol 2004; 44(2):66-70 (Abstract).

265. Ohman C, Imhof M, Roher HD. Trends in peptic ulcer bleeding and surgical treatment. World J Surg 2000; 24(3):284-293.

266. Odero W, Khayesi M, Heda PM. Road traffic injuries in Kenya: magnitude, causes and status of intervention. Inj Control Saf Promot 2003;10:53-61.

267. Oh DS, Pisegna JR. Management of upper gastrointestinal bleeding. Clin Fam Pract 2004; 6(3):631-645.

268. Okan A, Simsek I, Akpmar H, Ellidokuz E, Sanul AR, Aksoz K. Somatostatin and ranitidine in the treatment of non-variceal upper gastrointestinal bleeding: a prospective, randomized, double-blind, controlled study. Hepatogastroenterology. 2000;47:1325-7.

269. Palmer K.R. et al. British Society of Gastroenterology Endoscopy Committee. Non-variceal upper gastrointestinal hemorrhage: guidelines // Gut. 2002. -Vol. 51 (SupplIV); P. 1-6.

270. Papatheodoridis GV, Papadelli D, Cholongitas E, Vassilopoulos D, Mentis A, Hadziyannis SJ. Effect of Helicobacter pylori infection on the risk of upper gastrointestinal bleeding in users of nonsteroidal anti-inflammatory drugs. Am J Med 2004; 116(9):601-605.

271. Park CH, Sohn YH, Lee WS et al. The usefulness of endoscopic hemoclipping for bleeding Dieulafoy lesions. Endoscopy 2003; 35: 388-92.

272. Pavey DA, Craig PI. Endoscopic therapy for upper-GI vascular ectasias. Gastrointest Endosc. 2004; 59(2):233-8.

273. Paspalis GA,Matrella H, Kapsoritakis. A.Leontithis C,Papanikolao N, Chlouverakis GJ, Kouromalis E: An epidemilogical study of acute upper gastrointestinal bleeding in Crwete, Greece. Eur J Gasrroenterol Hepatol 2000; 12 (11): 1215-20.

274. Peden M, McGee, Sharma G. The injury chartbook. A graphical overview of the Global Burden of Injuries (Geneva: World Health Organization of 2002).

275. Pilotto A. Aging and upper gastrointestinal disorders. Best Pract Res Clin Gastroenterol.

2004;18:73-81.

276. Perez J., Dellinger R.P. Other Supportive therapies in sepsis // Intens. Care Med. 2001. - Vol.27, No.2. - P. 116-127.

277. Rajan R, Dhar P, Praseedom RK, Sudhindran S, Moorthy S. Role of contrast CT in acute lower gastrointestinal bleeding. Dig Surg 2004; 21:293-296.

278. Rios A, Montoya MJ, Rodriguez JM, Parrilla P. Emergency surgery in severe lower gastrointestinal hemorrhage. Cir Esp 2005; 78:308-311.

279. Ripoll *C,* Banares R, Beceiro I, et al. Comparison of transcatheter arterial embolization and surgery for treatment of bleeding peptic ulcer after endoscopic treatment failure. J Vasc Interv Radiol. 2004; 15(5):447-50

280. Ritz M.A., Frazer R., Tam W., Dent J. Impacts and patterns of disturbed gastrointestinal function in critically ill patients // Gastroenterol. 2000. - Vol.95.-P.3044-3052.

281. Ruiz B., Garay J., Correa P. Fontham E.T.H.. Morphometric evaluation of gastric antral atrophy: improvement after Helicobacter pylori // A JG., 2001. -Vol. 96. № 12. - P.3281-3287.

282. Sanders DS, Perry MJ, Jones SGW, Farlane E, Johnson AG, Gleeson DC, Lobo AJ. Effectiveness of an upper-gastrointestinal haemorrhage unit: a prospective analysis of 900 consecutive cases using the Rockall score as a method of risk standardization. Eur J Gastroenterol Hepatol 2004; 16:487494.

283. Sanders DS. Prospective validation of the Rockall risk scoring system for upper GI hemorrhage in subgroups of patients with varices and peptic ulcers. Am J Gastroenterol 2002; 97(3):630-635 (Abstract).

284. Sapoznikov B, Vilkin A, Hershkovici M, Fishman M, Eliakim R, Niv Y. Minidose aspirin and gastrointestinal bleeding: a retrospective case-control study in hospitalized patients. Dig Dis Sci. 2005 Sep; 50(9): 1621-4.

285. Savides TJ, Jensen DM. Therapeutic endoscopy for nonvariceal gastrointestinal bleeding. Gastroenterol Clin North Am. 2000; 29: 465-487

286. Schmulewitz N,Baillie J.Dieulafoy Lesions: A review of 6 years of experience at a territory referral center. Am J Gastroenterol. 2001;96:1688- 1694.

287. Schoenberg MH. Surgical therapy for peptik ulcer and nonvariceal bleeding. Langenbecks Arch Surg 2001; 386: 98-103.

288. Seewald S, Seitz U, Thonke F, et all. Interventional endoscopic treatment of upper

gastrointestinal bleeding-when,how, and how often. Langenbecks Arch Surg 2001; 386:88-97.

289. Sepulveda AR, Graham DY. Role of Helicobacter pylori in gastric carcinogenesis. Gastroenterol Clin North Am 2002;31: 517-35.

290. Seves I, Sousa C, Luz Z. Prognostic value of the finding of blood/ clots in the stomach at the emergency upper endoscopy. Acta Med Port 2002;15:413-416.

291. Shan L., Emanuel R.L., Dewald D., Torday J.S., Asokanathan N., Wada K., Wada E. and M.E.Sunday Bombesin-like peptide receptor gene expression, requlation, and function in fetal murine lung. Am.J.Physiol Lung Cell Mol Physiol, January 1, 2004; 286 (1): L165-173

292. Sharara AI, Rockey DC. Gastroesophageal variceal hemorrhage. N Engl J Med. 2001; 30: 345: 669-81.

293. Shirin H, Frenkel D, Shevah O, Levine A, Bruck R, Moss SF, Niv Y, Avni Y. Effect of proton pump inhibitors on the continuous real time (13)C-urea breath test. Am J Gastroenterol 2003;98:46-50.

294. Simoens M, Rutgeerts P. Non-variceal upper gastrointestinal bleeding. Best Pract Res Clin Gastroenterol 2001;15:121-33.

295. Skok P, Skok M. Upper Gastrointestinal tract hemorrhage and nonsteroidalantiinflamatory drugs- A 5-year prospective study. Zdrav Vestn 2002;71:153-6.

296. Sokic-Milutinovic A, Krstic M, Popovic D, et al. Role of Helicobacter pylori infection and use of NSAIDs in the etiopathogenesis of upper gastrointestinal bleeding. Acta Chir Iugosl 2007; 54: 51-62.

297. Spiegel BM. Endoscopy for acute nonvariceal upper gastrointestinal tract hemorrhage: is sooner better? A systematic review. Arch Intern Med 2001; 161(11):1393-1404 (Abstract).

298. Sung JJY. The role of acid suppression in the management and prevention of gastrointestinal hemorrhage associated with gastroduodenal ulcers. Gastroenterol Clin North Am 2003; 32(3):11-23.

299. Stollman N., Matz D.C. Pathophisiology and prophilaxis of stress ulcer in intensive care unit patients // J. Critical Care. Critical Care. 2005. - Vol. 20. P.35-45.

300. Tangmankongworakoon N. Results of emergency gastroscopy for acute upper gastrointestinal bleeding outside official hours at King Chulalongkorn Memorial Hospital J Med Assoc Thai 2003; 86(2):465-471 (Abstract).

301. Targownik LE, Gralnek IM, Dulai GS, Spiegel BM, Oei T, Bernstein CN. Management of acute nonvariceal upper gastrointestinal hemorrhage: a comparison of an American and a Canadian medical

center. Can J Gastroenterol. 2003 August; 17(8): 489-95.

302. Tashima K., Fujita A., Takeuchi K. Aggravation of ischemia/reperfusion-induced gastric lesions // Life Sci. 2000. Aug. 25. V. 67. № 14. P. 1707 - 1718.

303. Tew K, Davies RP, Jadun CK, Kew J. MDCT of acute lower gastrointestinal bleeding. AJR Am J Roentgenol 2004; 182:427-430.

304. Thiefin G, Jolly D. Impact of Helicobacter pylori infection on the risk of gastroduodenal ulcer in patients treated with non-steroidal anti-inflammatory drugs. Gastroenterol Clin Biol 2004;3:C45-57

305. Thomas C, Roland V. Can risk stratification improve the management of acute uppergastrointestinal bleeding. Eur J Gastroenterol Hepatol 2002; 14(5):475-476.

306. Thomopoulos KC, Vagenas KA, Vagianos CE, Margaritis VG, Blikas AP, Katsakoulis CE, Nikolopoulou VN. Changes in aetiology and clinical outcome of acute upper gastrointestinal bleeding during the last 15 years. Eur J Gastroenterol Hepatol 2004; 16:177-182.

307. Triadafilopoulos G. Reveew article: the role of antisecretory therapy in the management of non-variceal upper gastrointestinal bleeding //Aliment. Pharmacol. Ther. 2005. - Vol.22, No.3 - P.53-58.

308. van Leerdam ME, Vreeburg EM, Rauws EA, et al. Acute upper GI bleeding: did anything change? Time trend analysis of incidence and outcome of acute upper GI bleeding between 1993/1994 and 2000. Am J Gastroenterol. 2003; 98(7):1494-9

309. W.P.ter Beek, E.S.Muller, R.A.van Hoqezand, I.Biemond, and C.B.H.W. Lamers Gastrin releasing peptide reseptor expression is decreased in patients with Crohn's disease but not in ulcerative colitis. J.Clin, Pathol., October 1,2004; 57 (10): 1047-1051

310. Wolfe M.M., Sachs G. Acid suppression: Optimizing therapy for gastroduodenal healing, gastroesophageal reflux disease, and stress-related erosive syndrome // Gastroenterology. 2000. V. 118. P. 9-31.

311. Zheng K., Wu G., Cheng N.N., Yao C.J., Zhou L.F.. High risk factors of upper gastrointestinal bleeding affer neurosurgical procedures // Zhonghua Yi Xue ZaZhi. 2005. Vol.85, №48. - P.3387-3391.

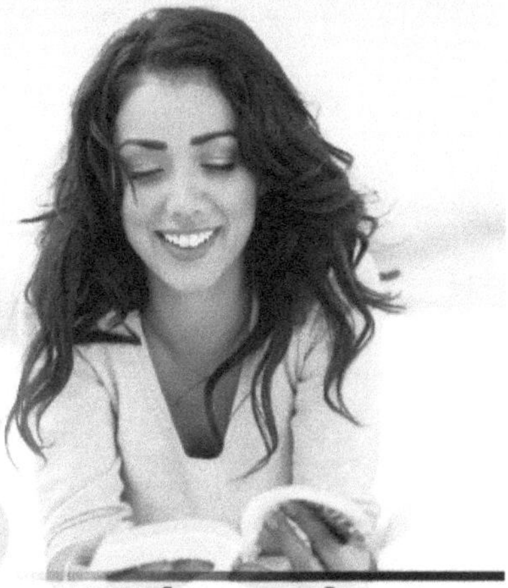

Kolibri 360 GmbH
Ferdinand-Jühlke-Straße 7
99095 Erfurt, Deutschland
produktsicherheit@kolibri360.de

Druck:
CPI Druckdienstleistungen GmbH
im Auftrag der
Kolibri 360 GmbH
Ferdinand-Jühlke-Str. 7
99095 Erfurt